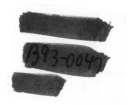

D1226347

A Colour Atlas of

Rheumatology

Third Edition

Michael Shipley
MA, MD, FRCP
Consultant Rheumatologist
Bloomsbury Rheumatology Unit
The Middlesex Hospital
London

Wolfe Publishing

Copyright © 1993 Mosby–Year Book Europe Limited.
Third edition published in 1993 by Wolfe Publishing, an imprint of Mosby–Year Book
Europe Limited
First edition 1974
Second edition 1980
Printed by BPCC Hazells Ltd, Aylesbury, England

ISBN 0 7234 1689 3

A CIP catalogue record for this book is available from the British Library.

For full details of all Mosby–Year Book Europe Limited titles, please write to Mosby–Year
Book Europe Limited, Brook House, 2–16 Torrington Place, London WC1E 7LT, England.

Contents

Dedication

This Third Edition is dedicated to all those people I have met who cope courageously with their chronic pain and disability.

Preface

This Third Edition seeks to contine the tradition begun by Dr Boyle of describing both the common and some of the rarer rheumatic diseases, using a series of clinical photographs, X-rays and histological pictures. The original captions have been replaced by text to enhance the value of the pictorial material and to allow description of the clinical presentation and management of these disorders.

In recent years, there have been major advances in the understanding of the immunology and genetics of rheumatic disorders, and this progress continues apace. The powerful tool of molecular biology is likely to make its mark on rheumatology in the next decade. At present, specific tests are helpful in making a diagnosis or in establishing a prognosis in some diseases, and thus in planning the treatment regime. However, understanding of the causes of many of these disorders remains poor. Despite this relative lack of knowledge, much can be done to alleviate the symptoms, if not to cure some of the diseases. It should be remembered that although many of the more common soft tissue and mechanical disorders are self-limiting, their outcome and the patient's speed of recovery can often be improved.

The diagnostic tools available to the rheumatologist include a wide variety of new imaging techniques; computed tomography (CT) and magnetic resonance imaging (MRI) have been developed since the publication of the Second Edition, and examples of both are now presented. Availability and cost continue to limit their use, and research is still needed to clarify exactly when such techniques provide valuable additional information and when their use is unnecessary and a waste of money.

Although these powerful investigative tools are available, rheumatology is an essentially clinical speciality. Skilled examination of the locomotor system is not difficult, but it is still not widely practised. In this Atlas, a simplified examination technique is described, highlighting what should be looked for in relation to specific joints.

Careful physical examination of the patient is an essential part of good practice. However, asking the right questions is the key to obtaining a good clinical history from the patient, and only on the basis of this history can the physical examination be carried out properly. In fact, in many cases the diagnosis can be made from the history alone, the physical examination being used primarily to clarify the differential diagnosis. Thus, a clear understanding of how the problems manifest themselves and of how patients are likely to describe them is fundamental. The art of listening and of sensitive questioning is too little taught, but it is essential to the proper practice of medicine, especially rheumatology. An understanding of the impact of social, psychological, environmental and cultural variations on the various diseases and their presentation is also vital, but takes practice to acquire. It is from the patients themselves that most is to be learnt.

In this edition there is a new section on the more common soft tissue problems that present to the rheumatologist, and some of the injection techniques that might be employed in their management are illustrated. As patients with rheumatic disorders may require surgical help for their disabilities and/or a variety of aids to enable them to lead as independent a life as possible, Chapters 11 and 12 introduce both the surgical management of chronic arthritis and some of the aids available.

It is hoped that this Atlas, with its accessible visual format, will be read not only by clinical medical students and doctors-in-training, but also by family practitioners and generalists. With an ever widening range of care teams involved in the treatment of patients with rheumatic disorders, it is also intended to be of value to physiotherapists, occupational therapists, nurses and other carers.

Acknowledgements

I am grateful to my colleagues in the Bloomsbury Rheumatology Unit at The Middlesex Hospital, particularly Drs Mary Corbett, Michael Snaith, David Isenberg and Jo Edwards for their advice and for allowing me access to their slide collections. Dr Michael Ehrenstein took some of the photographs The help of colleagues in other departments of the University College and Middlesex School of Medicine was invaluable in collecting many of the new illustrations. In particular, thanks are due to Drs Malcolm Chapman, Bill Lees and Margaret Hall-Craggs for their help with the imaging illustrations, Mr Jonathan Brazier for some of the ophthalmological slides, Professors Neville Woolf and Guy Nield, and Dr Mark Smith for histological slides, Professor David Easty for Figure 104, Dr Anthony Kurtz for Figures 284, 285, 307 and 308, and Dr Rob Miller for Figures 276 and 277. Dr Gerald Levene has generously allowed me to use Figures 224, 241 and 243–245 from his excellent *Colour Atlas of Dermatology* (Wolfe Publishing) and Figures 9, 10, 20, 21, 126, 269 and 270 are taken from the late Professor Lipman Kessel's *A Colour Atlas of Clinical Orthopaedics* (Wolfe Publishing). Dr Mike Bayliss loaned Figures 117 and 118, Dr Eric Hamilton provided Figure 316 , Mr Muirhead Allwood Figure 362, and Dr Andrew Keat Figure 209. I owe special thanks to Dr Barbara Ansell for her generous help and advice, and for providing most of the illustrations for the chapter on arthritis in childhood and allowing me to use others from her *Colour Atlas of Paediatric Rheumatology* (Wolfe Publishing). Figures 2, 34, 45 and 348 are taken from *Pocket Picture Guides to Clinical Medicine: Rheumatic Diseases,* published by Gower Medical Publishing and reproduced with their permission.

Finally, I would like to record my gratitude to the patients who have been pictured here and to the many others who have taught me much of what I know about the rheumatic disorders described in this book.

Michael Shipley

1 Introduction

Rheumatic complaints are common. Many soft tissue lesions and injuries are self-limiting and require little medical attention, recovering with the passage of time and with simple measures, such as rest, ice packs or bandaging. Such measures are often initiated instinctively by patients, drawing on their own knowledge or that of family and friends. One danger of a highly sophisticated and medicalised society is that such transient disorders are overinvestigated and then overtreated.

Patients frequently fear that symptoms of pain and stiffness, particularly if recurrent, imply a future of disability. Although these fears are sometimes well grounded, more often than not they are unjustified. For some, the anxiety may become a symptom in itself. Stress and anxiety are predominant features of modern life for many people, often playing a part in the persistence of a larger number of the common spinal muscular disorders. They contribute to increased muscular spasm and thus perpetuate pain. Stress also reduces the patient's ability to cope with the symptoms and their effects. The end result is that a vicious circle is set up: pain gives rise to stress and anxiety which, in turn, produces further pain, probably by inducing muscle spasm. A careful psychosocial history is often just as important as the results of blood tests or X-rays in planning the patient's management and thereby determining the outcome of the treatment. The aim of management of such patients is to exclude any major underlying disease, a process that requires a sound knowledge and understanding of locomotor disorders and general medicine, and then to give reassurance and explanation.

At the other end of the spectrum are the chronic disorders which may lead patients to life-long dependency on the medical profession, other health and social care professionals and on family and friends. Such patients need expert specialist help.

In between the two extremes lies a wide range of patients, some of whom can easily be dealt with by the interested generalist; others are best managed, or at least reviewed from time to time, by a rheumatologist.

A variety of clinical disorders may present with solely or predominantly rheumatic symptoms such as pain, stiffness, swelling or weakness. Certain of these disorders may be serious and potentially life-threatening, for example, the polymyalgic presentation of a patient with infective endocarditis, the myositic presentation of an underlying malignancy, a local primary or secondary bone tumour presenting as a monarthritis or spinal pain, osteomalacia presenting as bone pain, or an infective arthritis as a presenting symptom of AIDS. The list is long. The aim of this book is to describe both the simple and the more complex disorders, using carefully annotated clinical pictures.

The fascination of rheumatology lies in its diversity and in the essentially clinical skills upon which it depends. Yet it remains under-represented in the curricula of many medical schools and there is a low level of understanding among practising doctors of the often simple processes of examination and diagnosis of locomotor disorders. Some rheumatic diseases are readily curable or at least manageable; others are less so, but it is never the case that 'nothing can be done', an inaccurate statement made by doctors, health care professionals or friends, which is still too often repeated by arthritic patients. The myth that the lack of a cure for arthritis means that nothing helpful can be done must be dispelled and replaced by a positive approach that offers patients with locomotor disorders hope and, where appropriate, specialist care. Failing this, patients cannot be blamed for turning to complementary forms of medicine, some of which may be appropriate, while others are potentially disastrous.

History-taking and examination in disorders of the locomotor system

Examination of the locomotor system is a sadly neglected art. For all medical students, techniques for the examination of the chest, cardiovascular system, abdomen and neurological system are regularly reinforced, but examination of the joints is not routinely practiced. Indeed, most of the major general medical textbooks and many clinicians exclude the joints from their routine examination procedure. This is a shameful reflection of the fact that few senior clinicians have any idea of how to perform what is an essentially simple procedure.

History-taking

History-taking from patients with rheumatological disorders must include an initial discussion of the nature of the problem and of its impact on day-to-day life. The doctor will then need to direct and focus the discussion. Sometimes patients will have scoured their past in an attempt to understand why they are experiencing their current symptoms. Although this can be helpful, it may be necessary to guide them gently but firmly away from irrelevant historical facts and on to aspects of the problem that will help to establish the diagnosis. This involves inquiring about the nature, site and distribution of any pain or stiffness, the mode of onset (whether traumatic or without obvious cause) and the effect of activity and rest on the symptoms (rest often eases symptoms in mechanical disorders, but increases pain and stiffness in inflammatory processes), together with any other factors that may worsen or relieve the symptoms. Thus, in the differential diagnosis of pain in the neck, shoulder and arm, it is essential to decide whether it is neck or shoulder movements that exacerbate the pain. Associated sensory symptoms such as pins and needles (paraesthesia), numbness or weakness indicate that the pain is probably of neurological origin and may be due to a disc prolapse or nerve entrapment. In addition, the patient may have noticed that the joint symptoms are associated with localised swelling or redness, even though it may not be present at the time of the examination.

A brief general enquiry about the patient's state of health may indicate that the problem is part of a systemic disorder or a complication of a disorder that is not primarily rheumatological. Any previous similar episodes are relevant. A family history of similar complaints may give a clue if one of the inheritable disorders, such as gout or certain of the autoimmune diseases, is present. Specific enquiries about problems that are associated with the seronegative spond-arthritides (iritis, psoriasis, nonspecific urethritis, etc. – *see* Chapter 6) are important in the differential diagnosis of a polyarthritis. A drug history is essential and may, for example, indicate the cause of gout in an elderly woman taking diuretics (*see* p.59) or that of a lupus-like syndrome in a patient taking hydralazine or certain other drugs (*see* p.92).

When investigating the social history, the impact of the problem on the patient's working and family life should be clarified. There may be a direct link with the type of work performed or with an industrial injury, which may or may not be the subject of litigation. The patient's state of mind is important, be it relaxed or anxious: recent tragedy, loss of a job, or other stress or worry may be relevant to the cause of the problem itself, to the way in which the patient is coping with it, or to the timing of its presentation for medical attention. It is not uncommon for a complaint of pain, usually due to some relatively minor physical problem, to be the means by which a patient gains access to the doctor, with hopes of discussing other more complex and less easily verbalised problems such as family stresses or other anxieties. It is important that this is recognised and the patient is given the chance to talk.

Finally, it is helpful to ask the patient what they think might be the cause of their symptoms. Sometimes they are correct; at other times inappropriate fears may need to be dispelled.

A rapid examination of the locomotor system

Although full examination of the locomotor system and notation of the findings is time-consuming, it is possible to perform a rapid but thorough survey of the joints and their function, thereby localising those areas that require closer attention. The patient should first be asked if there is pain or stiffness in any particular joint or part of the spine.

In the course of the general locomotor examination it is important to ask the patient to mention any new or increased pain. During each movement, any loss of the normally smooth action should be noted as it usually indicates a local problem. The ranges of movement of the spine and joints must be related to the age of the patient (most stiffen as they age) and to genetic and racial origin (*see* **Hypermobility syndrome** p.135). The examination should always be directed by the information obtained from the history, and, if time is short or the problem is clearly localised, the examination can be limited to the limb or the part of the spine that the patient complains about, although this is not ideal. Where possible, patients should undress to their underwear to facilitate the detection of any swelling or other signs of inflammation, and of deformity or muscle wasting.

To examine the **upper limb**, patients should be observed as they make a series of simple movements. They should be instructed to:

- Raise both arms sideways straight up into the air (abduction).
- Then put both hands behind the neck and as far down the back as they can reach (external rotation in elevation).
- Finally, reach behind the back and as far up as possible (internal rotation in extension).

These three quick movements indicate any loss of shoulder movement or any pain arising from the shoulder or its rotator cuff.

- Hold the arms forwards with the elbows as straight as possible and the fingers spread apart.

Any fixed flexion at the elbow, with or without pain, implies a local problem. The hand and fingers can be examined for swelling, muscle wasting and deformity.

- Place the hands together in the 'prayer position' and then attempt to push the elbows as far up and out as possible.

Any flexion deformity of the fingers, whether it is due to joint, tendon or skin disease, can be seen with the hands in the prayer position. Pain or restriction of dorsiflexion of the wrist will limit the ability to raise the elbow(s) up and out.

- Make a tight fist with the thumbs held in the palm and then extend the fingers, palm upwards.

This indicates any loss of full flexion of the fingers, whatever the cause. If loss of flexion is found, function must be assessed carefully and the palmar aspect of the hand should be examined and palpated.

To examine the **lower limb**, patients should be instructed to:

- Walk a short distance away from and towards the observer.
- Sit down and rise from a chair without using their arms.
- Stand still, both facing and with the back to the observer.

This series of observations permits examination of the normal posture of all the joints of the lower limb while they are bearing weight and during walking, as well as a functional examination of the knees and hips under the stress of sitting down and getting up. A limp is always significant. Difficulties may arise from pain,

deformity, instability, weakness or any combination of these in one or more joints. Thus, walking with a bent knee may be due to: pain; swelling due to synovitis and/or an effusion of the hip or knee; or a fixed flexion deformity of the hip or knee or both. (Fixed flexion of the hip requires walking with a flexed knee in order to maintain the centre of gravity over the foot.)

- Attempt, while seated, to place one foot and then the other on the opposite thigh, keeping the back against the chair.

This is a sensitive test of pain arising from the hip, which is felt in the groin and the front of the thigh during the movement. Because it requires that the hip be both flexed and externally rotated, it also detects early loss of hip movement. Pain over the greater trochanter during this manoeuvre is likely to be due to a local trochanteric bursitis (*see* **343**) or, occasionally, to a problem originating in the lumbar region. If an abnormality is detected, a full examination of the hip should always be performed with patients lying on their back; loss of internal rotation in flexion is often the earliest sign of hip disease.

- Again while seated, attempt to straighten and flex the knees.

If the knees are abnormal, they *must* be examined with patients lying on their back and with the quadriceps muscle relaxed (*see* **39** and **40** for further details of examination for a knee effusion).

- Move each ankle up and down fully and then move each foot into inversion and eversion.
- Stand to permit examination of the weight-bearing position of the ankles, medial arches and toes.

If any pain or limitation is detected during this assessment, closer examination will be necessary, and formal testing of power, sensation and reflexes may be required. Any painful or abnormal joint should be palpated for warmth (indicating inflammation) and for swelling. The nature of any swelling, be it bony, 'boggy' (a term used to indicate the slight sense of give in swelling associated with synovial thickening) or due to a synovial effusion, should be determined, and a note made of any abnormal resting position or instability. The passive range of joint movement, which may differ from the active range, especially with certain problems arising from the tendons, should also be assessed.

To examine the **spine**, the whole of the back and the neck should be observed from behind. Instruct patients to:

- Attempt to bend forwards to touch the toes with the knees straight, to extend backwards and finally to run the hands down the lateral aspect of each thigh to the knee.
- Attempt to look over each shoulder, to put the chin on the chest and to look up to the ceiling.

This series of observations permits the spine to be viewed both at rest and during movement, demonstrating which manoeuvres are restricted or exacerbate pain. Any visible lateral curvature of the spine with a rotational component may be due to a primary scoliosis. This is often observed first in the teens or early twenties, and it is best seen from behind, with the patient bending forwards: the rotational element will be apparent as a prominence of one side of the rib cage. A secondary curvature may be due to degenerative disease in older patients, to inequality of leg length, or to muscle spasm induced by the acute pain of, for example, an acute lumbar disc prolapse. Curvature due to inequality of leg length or to muscle spasm will usually decrease or disappear when the patient is sitting or lying down.

- With the patient supine, the straight-leg-raising-test and femoral stretch tests are performed (*see* pp. 75 & 76). If the symptoms suggest an acute lumbar disc prolapse with nerve root irritation a full neurological examination is obligatory.

Palpation is frequently necessary in spinal disorders in order to detect localising factors, tender fibrositic nodules or trigger points (*see* Chapter 10).

Examination of the spine should include localisation of tender areas such as fibrositic nodules or trigger points, with the patient prone. In this position the sacro-iliac joints can also be stressed by pressure on the sacrum.

Using this rapid examination technique it is possible to exclude any major locomotor problem, or to localise it if one exists. It does not eliminate the need for a more exacting assessment if a specific abnormality is found. The pattern of joint and/or spinal involvement is important, as will become apparent in the following chapters.

2 Rheumatoid arthritis

Rheumatoid arthritis (RA) is the most common form of inflammatory arthritis and comprises the most constant element of the clinical workload of a rheumatologist because of the continuing patient care that it demands. It is a major cause of distress and disability from the mid thirties to old age. Certain types of postviral arthritis, particularly that which may follow rubella in adults, may mimic the onset of RA, although in such cases there is usually a typical history of the preceding viral illness or of contact with a known viral illness. It is important to recognise such postviral cases, since they remit in a few weeks or months and require only symptomatic treatment and reassurance.

RA usually affects the joints and periarticular structures most dramatically, and it is the resultant locomotor problems that have the greatest impact on the patient. It is, however, essentially a systemic disease, producing general symptoms of malaise, weight loss and anaemia, and it occasionally affects other organ systems. For this reason, it is frequently called rheumatoid disease.

The course of RA is unpredictable, with patients demonstrating a varying pattern of relapse and remission (**Table 1**). Although a small proportion of individuals develops severe disability relatively rapidly (chronic progressive RA), anxiety about this slight possibility must be balanced against the fact that as many as 25% of cases enter what appears to be a permanent remission, after a period of symptomatic disease which may last from 6 months to a few years (transient or remitting RA). Such cases can sometimes be recognised by the pattern of onset of symptoms and through the results of investigations.

Between the two extremes lies the majority of patients (persistent RA): these cases are afflicted at times by pain and stiffness of varying severity and have to try to adapt to living with this potentially disabling but rarely lethal disease. Risk factors that may indicate a worse-than-average prognosis include a gradual onset of synovitis, which affects an increasing number of joints over several weeks or months (rather than an acute onset of polyarthritis over a few days); being female; a family history of severe disease; possession of the HLA DR4 haplotype; a strongly and persistently positive rheumatoid factor level from the onset of symptoms; and the early development of bony erosions of the joints of the hands and feet, demonstrable on X-ray.

All patients with RA need specialist management. This management involves the judicious use of drugs, together with an appreciation of their potential benefits and side-effects, both of which are equally unpredictable. With increasing media interest in and public awareness of the possible risks of drug therapy, not only are clinical judgement and experience needed, but also good communication skills and a readiness to be frank about the risk of side-effects on the one hand, versus the risk of inaction in the face of a potentially devastating disease on the other. Equally important factors in management include advice from occupational therapists and physiotherapists about appropriate exercises and modifications to daily activities, which may reduce the load on the joint and diminish the risk of developing deformities.

Table 1. Clinical patterns of rheumatoid disease.

1 Palindromic
Attacks of 24–48 hours. 50% progress to patterns 3–5.
2 Transient
Self-limiting in <12 months. No permanent sequelae.
3 Remitting
Remission after 3–5 years. Minimal residual damage.
4 Persistent
Relapsing and remitting cases, with variable disability.
5 Chronic and progressive
Leads to severe deformity and disability.

Patients are often understandably depressed and anxious at the onset of RA, with all its implications for their future and that of their families. Sensitive and sympathetic handling is required, and the help of a psychologist or trained counsellor may be appropriate. Once the patient has been assessed by a rheumatologist, specially trained rheumatology nurses, where available, are helpful as a point of first referral for queries from patients. In systems where primary and specialist health care coexist, it is appropriate that care of RA patients should be shared. The primary health care team should provide week-to-week support, with intermittent visits to a specialist, whose exposure to a wider case load offers an experienced overview on drug management, the need for referral for specialist surgery, and the risk of developing complications.

Studies suggest varying prevalence of the disease. This is partly due to geographical population and genetic differences, but probably also reflects disparity in the ways in which the disease is defined and recorded. In most European and North American studies it appears that 0.5–1% of the population is affected. This figure is apparently lower in parts of the Middle East and Asia, although this may reflect under-recording. Climate does not appear to play a role, although it can modify the impact of the symptoms to some extent. RA can start at any age, from early childhood to extreme old age, but the incidence peaks between 30 and 50 years of age. The disease has a female preponderance, affecting premenopausal women in particular. In RA presenting for the first time in later life, the sexes are equally affected. The female preponderance has encouraged research on the possible role of sex hormones in the aetiology of the disease. Although not all studies agree, it appears that the use of the contraceptive pill during early reproductive life slightly reduces the risk of developing RA later. The observation that RA often goes into remission in the second and third trimesters of pregnancy has excited interest for over 60 years. Investigation of this phenomenon led to the discovery of the corticosteroid drugs, but it has still not produced a safe or certain therapeutic approach. The exact role of hormones in the onset or the modification of the disease process remains unclear.

Of further aetiological interest is the tendency of RA to run in families. Sporadic cases are common, but there is often a history of RA in a relative, particularly in cases of more severe disease. Studies of monozygotic twins suggest that genetic factors account for about 30% of the risk of developing RA. In northern European Caucasians there is a close association between RA and the tissue type HLA DR4. In Israeli and Indian populations the association is with HLA DR1. Indeed in northern Europe, DR4- and DR1-positive individuals represent 90–95% of cases of RA, almost equalling the striking hundred-fold increase in the relative risk of developing ankylosing spondylitis in the presence of HLA B27 (*see* p.77). A second, nonHLA DR-related genetic factor is almost certainly also present in these RA populations. In Spain, southern Italy and Greece there is no association with either DR1 or DR4, suggesting that a different disease variant exists in these populations.

Any aetiological theory for this complex disease must explain both its onset and its variable chronicity. Despite much dedicated research, a clear understanding has not emerged. That a viral or other antigenic trigger is involved, possibly lying dormant until tripped by some extrinsic or intrinsic event in an environment which is genetically and hormonally primed, is an attractive suggestion, but it has not been supported by the finding of any such triggers.

Whatever the cause of RA, the end result is a chronic inflammatory process (mainly restricted to the synovial membrane) which is autoimmune and apparently driven by a hidden antigen. It is the synovial inflammation that causes the pain, swelling and stiffness of active rheumatoid synovitis, and that may eventually lead to irreversible damage. The presence of large numbers of plasma cells in the synovium, some of which produce rheumatoid factors, suggests that they may play an important role in causing the chronicity of the inflammation. Activated macrophages and lymphocytes are also present, an observation which suggests an important role for cellular immune mechanisms and cytokines in the underlying process.

1 Schematic representation of rheumatoid factor. This diagram of an immunoglobulin molecule illustrates the basic structure. Two light and two heavy polypeptide chains are held together by disulphide bonds (S-S) to form a constant region (Fc) and a variable region (Fab). The variable sequences of peptides lead to the extraordinary variability of the antibody-combining sites. Rheumatoid factors are immunoglobulins, autoantibodies whose antigen is the Fc portion of human immunoglobulin itself. They are sometimes known as 'antiglobulins'. Cross-reactivity occurs with immunoglobulins from other species, a phenomenon which led Rose and Waaler, working independently in the 1930s and 1940s, to discover the existence of these rheumatoid factors. Both men demonstrated that sheep red cells, 'sensitised' by serum from a rabbit previously injected with sheep red cells, agglutinated when mixed with serum from certain patients with RA. It is now known that these 'sensitised' cells are coated with rabbit immunoglobulin (rabbit anti-sheep antibodies), with which the patient's antiglobulins react. A variety of tests specifically for human IgM rheumatoid factors is now available, most of which still depend upon agglutination of particles.

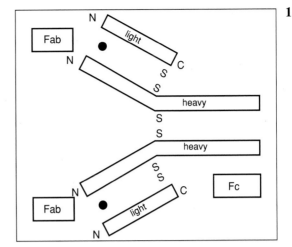

2 Latex agglutination test. Latex particles are coated with the Fc portion of human immunoglobulin and mixed with serial dilutions of the patient's serum. Patients with RA may also have IgA and IgG rheumatoid factors in their serum, which are detectable by different techniques. The presence of a titre of 1/40 (or less) of IgM rheumatoid factor is not significant; normal individuals, particularly older people, may have even higher levels. Chronic infections or other chronic inflammatory diseases may also lead to raised titres. *A positive rheumatoid factor test at any titre is not diagnostic of RA, although it may help to confirm a clinical diagnosis and aid prognostication.* A persistently high rheumatoid factor signifies a greater risk of more severe disease, although this is not invariable. There is some indication from population surveys that asymptomatic individuals with positive rheumatoid factors are slightly more at risk of developing RA at a later date than those with persistently negative rheumatoid factor tests.

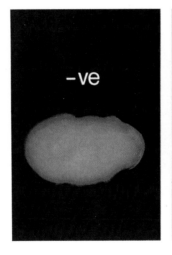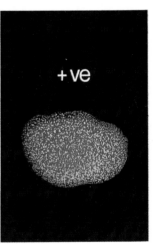

IgG antiglobulin monomer	Self-associated IgG antiglobulin complex

Fc

Antiglobulin binding site

3 Self-associating IgG rheumatoid factors. IgG rheumatoid factors are able to self-associate, as shown in this diagrammatic representation. The resultant immune complexes may combine with IgM rheumatoid factors in the joint and activate complement, thus stimulating and perpetuating the inflammatory cascade.

Pathology

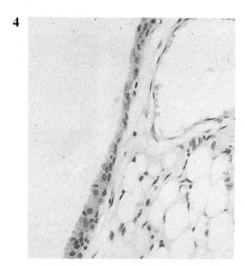

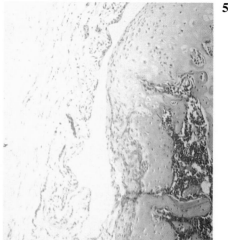

4 & 5 Normal synovium and early RA changes. The normal synovial membrane is a network of capillaries, venules and lymphatics lying in a loose, apparently unstructured and relatively acellular stroma of collagen fibres, which contains scanty fibrocytes. The surface layer is 1–3 cells thick and comprises phagocytes, cells which have a synthetic function and some pluripotential cells. 5 illustrates a finger joint with the synovial membrane (on the left) and the synovial angle and its reflection onto the periosteum. Normal cartilage and subarticular bone are also shown (on the right).

As early RA is not often seen by a specialist the earliest synovial changes are rarely biopsied. There is probably a flux of polymorphonuclear leucocytes from the extensive synovial vascular network, moving between the surface lining cells and into the synovial cavity. This is associated with increased vascular permeability, consequent synovial oedema and the development of a joint effusion. These changes are potentially reversible.

A similar mechanism is probably the basis of the acute episodes of joint pain and swelling seen in patients with **palindromic rheumatism**. This is an episodic monarthritis in which acute pain, swelling and redness flare and settle within a few days, only to reflare in another joint a few days, weeks or months later. During this phase of palindromic rheumatism, permanent joint damage does not occur. With time, about 50% of such patients go on to develop the more chronic synovitis typical of RA: conversion to seropositivity for rheumatoid factor is associated with an increased risk of developing a chronic, progressive arthritis.

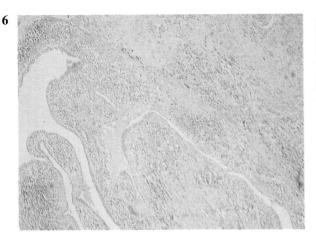

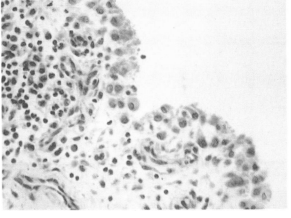

6 Synovium in RA. The reason for the chronicity of the inflammatory process in RA is not fully understood. The synovial tissue is hypertrophied and thrown up into multiple villi. There is massive infiltration with lymphocytes and plasma cells, and the stroma is fibrotic. Generally, a synovial biopsy from a patient with RA is indistinguishable microscopically from those from most other chronic inflammatory arthritides; it serves only to exclude infection or rarer causes of joint inflammation.

7 Synovium in RA (higher magnification). The synovium is oedematous, with separation of endothelial cells reflecting an active flux of cells into the stroma, which demonstrates infiltration with lymphocytes and plasma cells. There is proliferation of the synovial lining cell layer and of the stromal cells. Lymphocytes and plasma cells lie just beneath the synovial membrane. A significant proportion of the plasma cells produces rheumatoid factors locally and may thus contribute to the chronic inflammation.

8

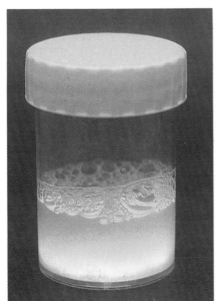

Table 2. Examination of synovial fluid.

Appearance		
	Clear	OA
	Cloudy or opalescent	Seronegative arthritis or RA
	Turbid	Crystal synovitis
	Purulent	Infection
	Haemorrhagic	Trauma (*see* p.123)
Cell count (using EDTA sample tube)	High cell count (>50,000) Predominance of polymorphs	} Cystal synovitis or infection
Gram stain and culture	Identification of infective organism Choice of antibiotic	
Microscopy under polarised light	Identification of crystals	

8 Inflammatory synovial fluid. The joint effusion is highly viscous. Its cloudy, opalescent appearance is due to increased cellularity. Dead and dying polymorphs and lymphocytes are the predominant cells seen on microscopy. The appearance of the fluid is helpful in distinguishing different types of arthritis but not diagnostic. A cell count is indicative but not specific. Gram staining and microscopy under polarised light may be diagnostic. **Table 2** indicates the likely diagnoses for the different observations made on synovial fluid.

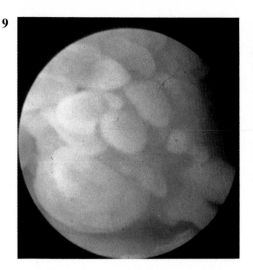

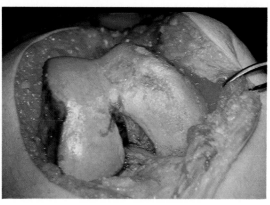

9 & 10 Arthroscopic and operative views of chronically inflamed synovium. In RA the normally smooth synovium is thickened and thrown up into folds and villi which project into the joint cavity and are easily visible on arthroscopy (**9**). This phase remains potentially reversible and X-rays appear normal or may show soft tissue swelling and juxta-articular osteoporosis.

If the inflammatory process continues unchecked, it causes irreversible damage and consequent disability. The inflammation extends beyond the synovial membrane to involve adjacent bone and cartilage, as well as soft tissue structures, such as tendons and the joint capsule. This type of damage is illustrated in the operative view (**10**) of a patient with long-standing RA. Not only is the synovium thickened and inflamed but the cartilage of the femoral condyles is ulcerated, and erosion of bone is apparent at the border of the medial femoral condyle. The damage itself causes symptoms and, when deciding on management, it is always important to distinguish between symptoms due to chronic inflammation and those due to its destructive end results (*see* **Treatment**, p.47).

11

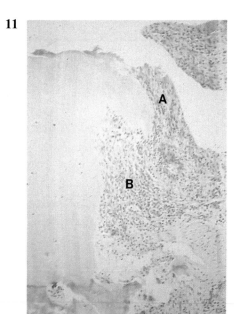

11 Synovial pannus (A) and early erosion (B). At the reflection of the synovial lining and capsule onto the bony periosteum, and at the margin of the articular cartilage, the inflamed and hypertrophied synovium expands across the cartilage surface, producing a pannus. The pannus impairs the normal nutrition of the cartilage from the joint space and chemically influences the chondrocytes via locally produced cytokines. This process leads to cartilage damage which, as it increases, thins the cartilage. The resultant joint space narrowing is visible on X-ray. The inflamed synovium may also infiltrate the cartilage and bone directly, leading to what is seen on X-ray as a typical rheumatoid juxta-articular erosion (*see* **25-27**).

Joint deformities may develop during this phase, due partly to the bone and cartilage changes, and partly to weakening and stretching of the joint capsule and associated tendons. Where the process continues unchecked, gross joint destruction develops in a small proportion of cases. Even if the inflammation eventually remits, the damage may progress due to the development of secondary osteoarthritis (*see* p.49).

12 Histology of a rheumatoid nodule. The most diagnostic of histological appearances in RA is the rheumatoid nodule. Nodules may occasionally form in the synovium and are the one diagnostic manifestation of RA if seen in a synovial biopsy. They most commonly develop subcutaneously over bony surfaces, typically on the ulnar surface of the forearm, but they may form anywhere (*see* **28, 29, 81 & 82**). Histologically, there are three zones: a central necrotic area, mainly composed of fibrin (at bottom of picture); a surrounding area in which histiocytes and fibroblasts form radiating columns or palisades; and an outer layer of chronic inflammatory infiltration, which contains variable numbers of fibroblasts.

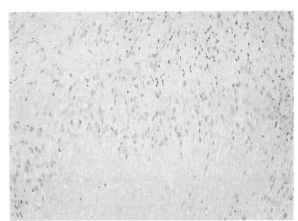
12

Articular and periarticular involvement

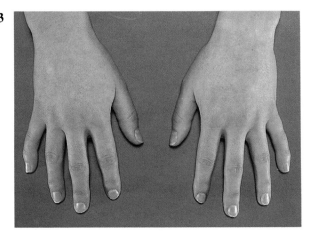
13

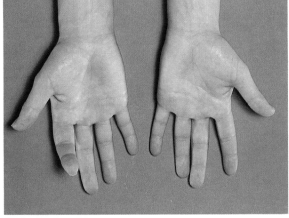
14

13 Early RA of the hands. RA usually presents as a symmetrical, peripheral, inflammatory arthritis of the small joints. The fingers are swollen and flexed owing to synovitis affecting the metacarpophalangeal (MCP) and proximal interphalangeal (PIP) joints of both hands. The distal interphalangeal (DIP) joints are typically spared. In addition to the swelling, the patient complains of pain and stiffness, which are worse in the morning. On examination the swelling does not feel hard, but firm or boggy. The swelling may feel fluctuant if an effusion is present. Even early in the course of the disease, involvement of finger joints and tendon sheaths is disabling and impairs many normal activities.

14 Tenosynovitis of the flexor tendons of the finger. Flexor tendon sheath synovitis may also cause finger stiffness. Here, it is most marked in the index finger of the right hand. The thickened tendons can be palpated in the palm. Tendon nodules may lead to 'triggering' of the finger: the patient awakens with the affected finger(s) stuck in the flexed position. This may also occur during a power grip. If the tenosynovitis is mild and the nodule small, the finger can be straightened with difficulty and, sometimes, with pain. If the problem is more severe, the finger becomes immovably flexed.

Extension of flexor tenosynovitis proximally and/or inflammation of the wrist joint may lead to carpal tunnel syndrome (*see* **106, 107, 339 & 340**).

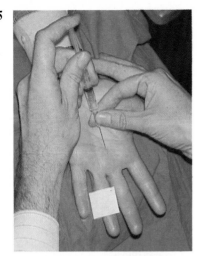

15 Injection technique for flexor tenosynovitis. The best treatment for flexor tenosynovitis is to inject a small volume of a local anaesthetic, followed by 0.2–0.5 ml of a semicrystalline preparation such as hydrocortisone hemisuccinate or triamcinolone hexacetonide, into the tendon sheath (not the tendon itself) in the palm, using a fine needle (*see* pp.145–146 for general guidance on injection techniques). Early treatment of finger flexor tenosynovitis is essential if later impairment of hand function is to be minimised. Carpal tunnel syndrome may require splinting, injection or surgical release (*see* **106, 107, 339 & 340**).

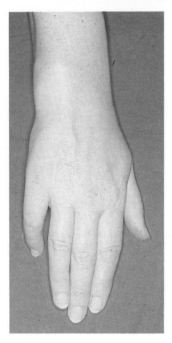

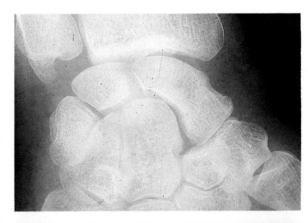

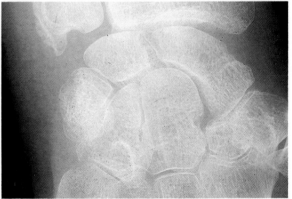

16–18 Early wrist involvement in RA. 16 shows the early clinical appearance. The ulnar styloid is often the site of early pain and swelling. Restriction of dorsiflexion and palmar flexion and of supination and pronation of the wrist may occur. The wrist feels weak. Frequently, the ulnar styloid is also the site of the earliest erosive changes visible on X-ray. Compare the ulnar styloid on the still normal wrist X-ray in **17** with that in the X-ray taken 4 years later (**18**): the styloid has become eroded and there is overlying soft tissue swelling. Several early erosions in the carpal bones are also present.

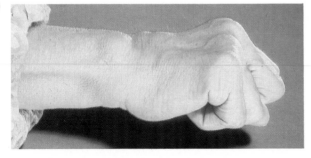

19 Dorsal tenosynovitis of wrist. The dorsal tendon sheath may be affected by synovitis, often producing a typical hourglass-shaped swelling. This shape is due to compression of the swollen sheath by the extensor retinaculum at the wrist.

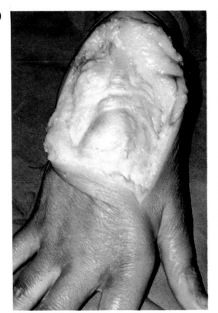

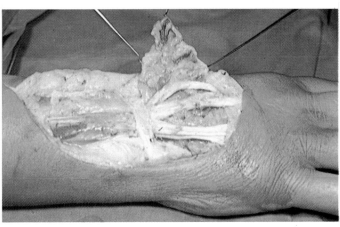

20 & 21 Dorsal tenosynovitis at the wrist. The hypertrophic extensor tendon sheaths have been exposed surgically and the extensor retinaculum can be seen (**20**). The chronically inflamed synovium can then be dissected away from the tendons (**21**).

22 & 23 Ruptured extensor tendons of the finger. The combination of an inflamed, eroded and dorsally subluxed ulnar styloid with dorsal extensor tenosynovitis may damage the extensor tendons of the fingers, causing rupture. The patient is unable to extend the affected finger(s) voluntarily. The little and ring fingers are the most frequently affected. To avoid disabling and permanent flexion deformities of the fingers, surgery within a few weeks is necessary. The tendons are often severely damaged, with the proximal ends retracted into the forearm. Repair is effected by tendon transfer from adjacent fingers. At the same time, surgical synovectomy of the wrist and excision of the ulnar styloid may be performed.

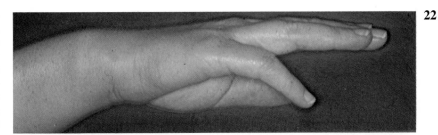

22

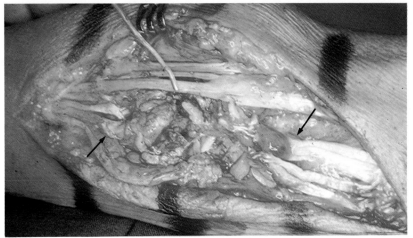

23

24

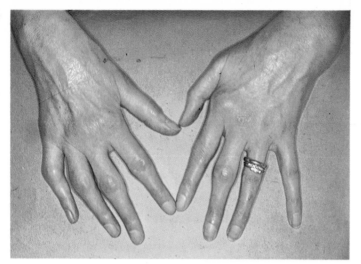

24 More advanced hand involvement in RA. In early disease, function can be severely impaired by pain and stiffness. However, if the disease process is controlled and these symptoms are reduced, function may return to normal. If the inflammation continues unchecked, more marked hand changes develop, and irreversible deformity and impaired function may result. Before deciding on the treatment, it is important to decide whether disability is due to active synovial inflammation, deformity, or both. Here, the left little finger is drifting into ulnar deviation. Other fingers may follow. This deformity is due to a combination of weakening of the MCP joint capsule and the natural 'ulnarwards' pull of muscles during power gripping. Such ulnar deviation, which is not necessarily severely disabling, is best managed with exercises and advice from an occupational therapist. The right little finger shows a flexion deformity at the PIP joint, which may reverse if the swelling reduces. However, it may be due to damage to the middle slip of the finger extensor, with herniation of the joint between the two collateral slips – a boutonnière deformity. An experienced hand surgeon may be able to prevent or delay the development of such deformities.

25

26

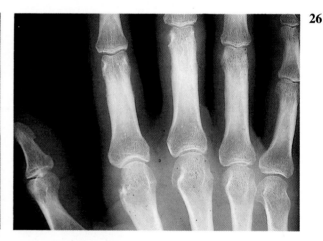

27

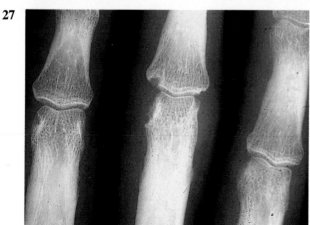

25–27 Erosion affecting the MCP and PIP joints. In this patient, progressive damage developed over a period of 6 years, with erosions and loss of joint space. The 1980 X-rays were normal, apart from soft tissue swelling around the PIP joint of the middle finger (**25**). By 1984, there was clear loss of cortical definition of the radial border of the index metacarpal head. Early erosions could also be seen around the PIP joint of the middle finger (**26**). The close-up film from 1986 (**27**) reveals how the early changes progressed around the PIP joint of the middle finger. The PIP joints of the index and little finger had also developed early erosions. Despite the fact that second-line drugs (see p.47) were started in 1984, they failed to arrest this progressive damage. However, between 1986 and 1991 little further damage occurred, except to the wrists.

Most rheumatologists believe that second-line drugs retard the erosive process, even if they do not halt it. Earlier more aggressive use of these drugs offers some hope of preventing the worst ravages of the disease. In addition, an increasing, highly specialised interest in hand surgery in rheumatoid arthritis is developing, which may help to prevent functional deterioration. Such surgery should not be undertaken by a general orthopaedic surgeon.

28

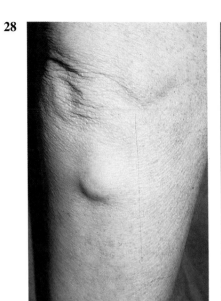

29

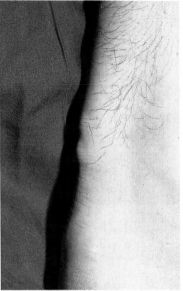

28 & 29 Rheumatoid nodules. These typical lesions of RA are usually subcutaneous, nodular, and firm (rather than hard or soft) on palpation. Rheumatoid nodules may occur at any stage of the disease, usually in patients who have a strongly positive rheumatoid factor test. They arise most commonly over pressure points such as the elbow (**28**) or the Achilles tendon (**29**), but may occur anywhere, especially in bed-bound patients (*see* **82**). Often asymptomatic, they can be painful on direct pressure and may cause ulceration of overlying skin (*see* **81**). Rheumatoid nodules can be excised, but they often recur. Spontaneous regression usually, but not invariably, accompanies effective drug-induced disease control or natural remission. Their appearance early in the course of the disease suggests a worse-than-average prognosis.

30 Early involvement of the feet. The metatarsophalangeal (MTP) joints may be affected early in the disease, producing painful metatarsalgia and swelling of the forefoot. The forefoot is painful when squeezed and the MTP joints are palpably swollen. Splaying of the toes, the 'daylight sign', is caused by this MTP joint swelling. In this patient the MTP joint of the second toe is swollen. Wider shoes with cushioned soles help.

30

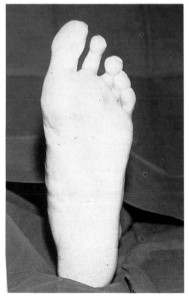

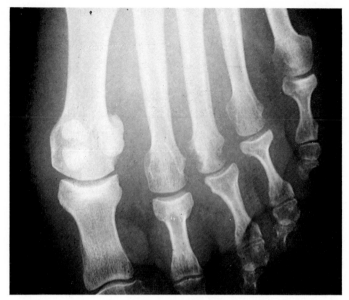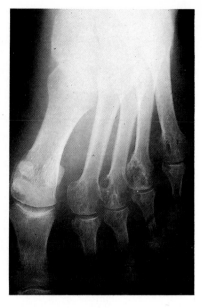

31 & 32 Early erosions of the MTP joints. In early inflammatory arthritis, even if the feet are asymptomatic but RA is suspected, X-rays of the feet may show diagnostic erosions of the metatarsal heads (**31**) before any are visible on hand X-rays. Such erosions indicate a need either to introduce second-line therapy or to review existing second-line therapy. In **32**, taken several years later, the erosive change is more extensive despite treatment.

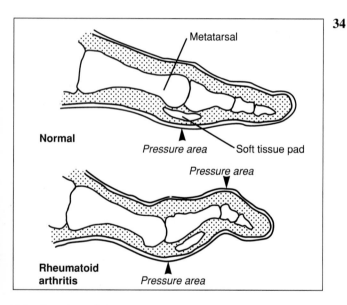

33 & 34 Established RA of the forefoot. In the rheumatoid forefoot the MTP joints sublux and the metatarsal heads become displaced towards the sole of the foot. The toes develop fixed flexion deformities (right foot). This combination destroys the normal relationship of the protective fibrofatty pad to the weight-bearing MTP joints, and the metatarsal heads become painful on weight-bearing. Secondary painful callosities on the sole of the foot are common and the hammered toes rub against the shoe upper, developing painful pressure points. Simultaneously, the MTP joint of the great toe frequently develops a valgus deformity, and shoewear produces increased pressure over the joint itself, leading to a painful and inflamed bursa or bunion. Special shoes to accommodate the feet and to distribute pressure more evenly over the sole are appropriate and may improve walking considerably. Despite recent improvements in style and design, the unattractive appearance of such shoes, cut to conform to the shape of the deformed foot, upsets many patients. Nonetheless, they increase comfort, may prevent secondary ulceration and should be encouraged for everyday use. A forefoot arthroplasty (*see* **35, 348 & 349**) is an effective procedure if pain persists.

35 Callosities complicating RA of the forefoot.
Callosities form over the subluxed metatarsal heads and make walking painful. There is a risk of secondary ulceration, which is an important potential source of septicaemia and thus of infection of other joints (*see* **64–68**); artificial replacements, even of remote joints, are particularly susceptible to secondary infection. A surgical forefoot arthroplasty (*see* **348 & 349**), excising the metatarsal heads and restoring the fibrofatty pad to its correct weight-bearing position, with correction of the hallux valgus if necessary, is appropriate when the pain is severe or if ulceration develops. This safe and effective procedure reduces pain but leaves the foot about half a shoe size smaller. Leading shoe manufacturers will provide unequally sized 'pairs' by special request.

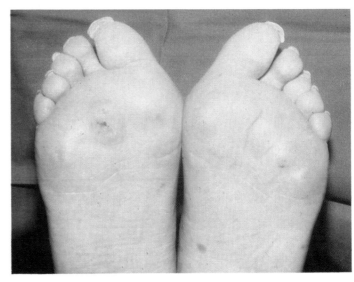

35

36 & 37 Hindfoot deformity in RA.
Involvement of the subtaloid and midtarsal joints leads to a valgus deformity of the hindfoot, with pain in these joints on weight-bearing. Slight wedging of the medial border of the heel of the shoe may help, but if hindfoot pain and instability are severe, a fusion of the subtaloid joint should be considered. This procedure requires that the foot bears no weight for several months, and the resultant need to use crutches may cause pain in other affected joints, particularly the shoulders and wrists. Both of the patients illustrated have severe hind- and midfoot damage, with total collapse of the medial arch and a valgus deformity of the hindfoot. Surgery will not help and special shoes will be of only limited benefit. In **36** a pressure sore is developing under a prominent bone in the midtarsal region. This will require careful attention to footwear and padding if it is to heal. The lifting of the subluxed toes from contact with the ground, clearly visible in both patients, is caused by metatarsal subluxation.

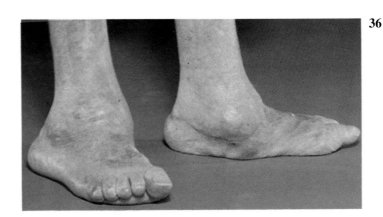

36

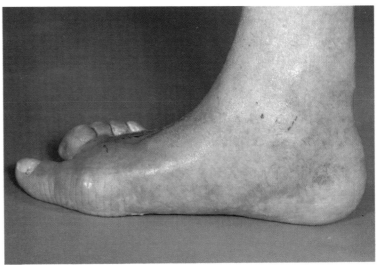

37

38

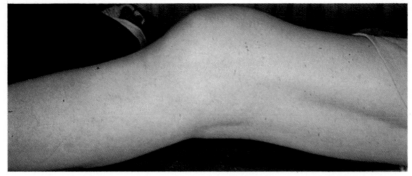

38 Synovitis of the knee. Although RA usually produces a symmetrical small joint arthritis, larger joints are often affected simultaneously. Up to 20% of patients present initially with a monarthritis of any joint, but most commonly it is the knee. Pain, stiffness and swelling are the presenting features. A fixed flexion deformity is common, especially where there is an effusion, and quadriceps muscle wasting rapidly ensues. On examination, the swelling fills in the parapatellar dimples and expands the suprapatellar pouch. The joint feels warm, differentiating it from the 'cool' synovitis of osteoarthritis or trauma.

39

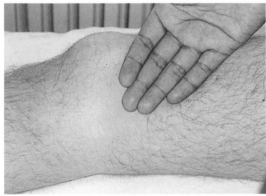

40

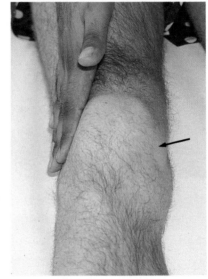

39 & 40 Bulge sign for a synovial effusion. An effusion may not be immediately apparent. It can be detected when the patient lies with the knee straight and the quadriceps muscle relaxed. A gentle sweeping pressure is exerted against the medial border of the joint (**39**). The medial dimple (**40**, arrow) is then observed while gentle pressure is applied on the lateral side of the joint. If an effusion is present, a slightly delayed bulging of the medial dimple is seen as the fluid is displaced medially.

If the effusion is large, insufficient fluid will be displaced from the medial compartment to see it bulging back. However, firm compression of the suprapatellar pouch by one hand, followed by firm and quick pressure on the patella from the front, results in a tapping sensation as the patella hits the femoral condyles. This tap is delayed when an effusion is present – a positive patellar tap sign. At the same time the proximal hand feels the fluid being forced back into the suprapatellar pouch.

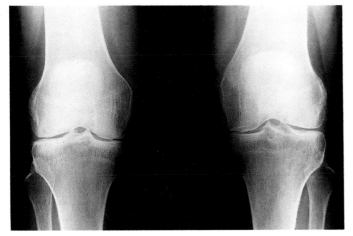

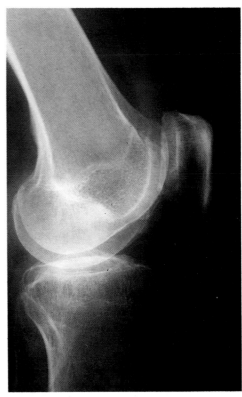

41 & 42 Established RA of the knee. When the knees are first affected, X-rays may be normal or show only soft tissue swelling. An effusion can be seen on this lateral view as a radiolucent area displacing the soft tissues away from the anterior surface of the femur (**42**). In the severely inflamed knee, the juxta-articular bone may become osteoporotic. Cartilage thickness is reduced in progressive RA, affecting one compartment or, as here, both equally. Erosions are uncommon in the knee. This patient had had RA for 4 years. Her knees were swollen and stiff, but mobility was still good. Contrast the lack of sclerosis and osteophyte formation in this inflammatory arthritis with that seen in typical osteoarthritis (OA) (*see* **130 & 132**).

43

44

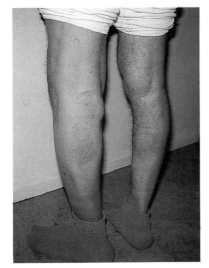

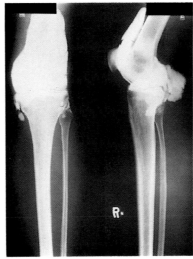

43 & 44 Popliteal cyst. Any effusion in the knee may be forced under pressure into the semimembranosus bursa in the medial popliteal fossa. In some patients this produces a painful swelling (here of the left knee), which may vary in size and tenseness with rest and walking. This is probably because the opening to the bursa acts as a valve, allowing fluid into the cyst but not back into the knee. The diagnosis is best confirmed by ultrasound or magnetic resonance imaging (MRI), techniques which, where available, have largely superseded the arthrogram. This arthrogram (**44**) demonstrates the cyst. The best treatment is to aspirate the knee joint (*see* **341**) and inject a cortico-steroid. (Aspiration and injection of the cyst itself is not recommended.) Ideally, the patient should rest as much as possible for a couple of days after the injection.

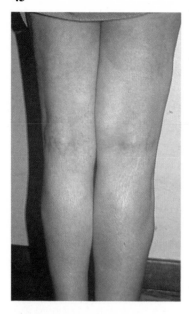 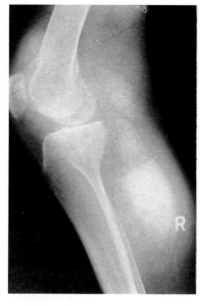 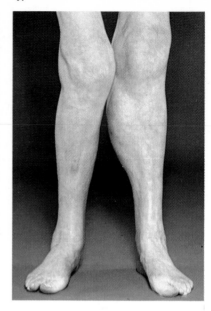

45 & 46 Ruptured popliteal cyst. Pressure in the cyst may cause it to rupture, producing the sensation of a sudden kick behind the knee, followed by pain and swelling of the calf, and oedema of the ankle. The appearance is strikingly like that of a deep venous thrombosis (DVT), with which it is commonly confused. A history of a previously swollen knee (no longer swollen, unless there is marked synovitis, because all the fluid is now in the calf), an acute onset, and pain that is worse high in the calf and in the popliteal fossa, rather than in the midcalf, are all helpful pointers. If in doubt, diagnostic ultrasound of the calf will distinguish a ruptured popliteal cyst from a DVT, and is preferable to arthrography or venography. The arthrogram demonstrates the leakage of fluid into the calf. Treatment is with bed rest, aspiration and injection of the knee and, if the pain is severe, with appropriate oral anti-inflammatory agents, not anticoagulants!

47 Advanced RA of the knees. This patient has valgus knees (more marked on his right) caused by lateral tibial plateau collapse. The hindfeet also show early valgus deformities (*see* **36 & 37**). In contrast, collapse of the medial tibial plateau would produce a varus deformity. The left calf is swollen by a huge cyst caused by a chronic, painless leak of synovial fluid from a ruptured popliteal cyst.

48 Advanced RA changes in the knee. Progressive rheumatoid damage to cartilage and bone has produced almost complete joint space loss in this weight-bearing film, taken while the patient is standing. There is also bony erosion and early collapse of the medial tibial plateau, producing a varus knee.

49 Tibial plateau collapse in RA. Weight-bearing on an eroded and osteoporotic tibial plateau can cause its collapse. This may happen insidiously, with gradual development of instability and deformity, but it may also occur acutely, with sudden pain and deformity. In this non weight-bearing film, taken with the patient lying down, the lateral tibial plateau has collapsed, leading to valgus deformity of the knee when weight-bearing (*see* **47**).

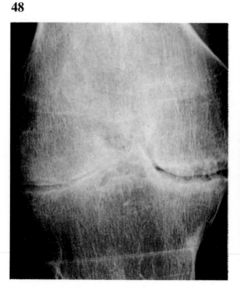 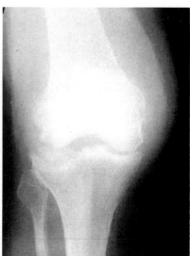

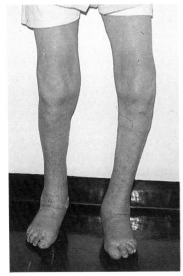
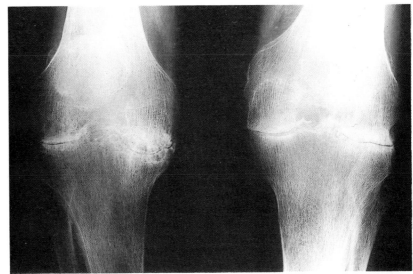

50–52 End-stage knees in RA. Patients may develop one valgus and one varus knee ('windswept' knees). There is dramatic loss of cartilage and damage to the underlying bone. With this degree of damage the only approach is to discuss the possibility of total knee replacement, a procedure which can both reduce pain and improve mobility (*see* **356**).

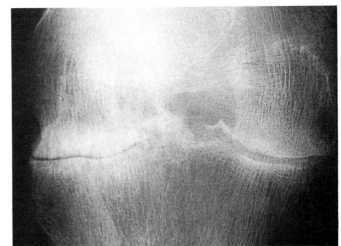

53 RA affecting the right hip. The hips are spared in many patients with RA, the most common cause of discomfort around the hip being trochanteric bursitis, which produces pain and tenderness over the greater trochanter. (Many patients mistake this for hip involvement and become unduly concerned.) A local corticosteroid injection into the point of maximum trochanteric tenderness (*see* **343**) will help.

When the hip joint itself is affected, the pain is felt in the groin, buttock and anterior thigh, and sometimes predominantly in the knee. (In any patient with knee pain, always examine the hip to exclude it as the primary source of the pain.) Clinically, the hip may be restricted in movement and the pain reproduced during clinical examination, either during movement or at the end of the range. At this stage, X-rays may be normal or they may demonstrate global joint space loss on the affected side, where there will be periarticular osteoporosis and none of the reactive sclerosis seen in primary or secondary OA (*see* **133–135**). Here, the right hip shows loss of joint space, with irregularity of the upper medial surface of the femoral head.

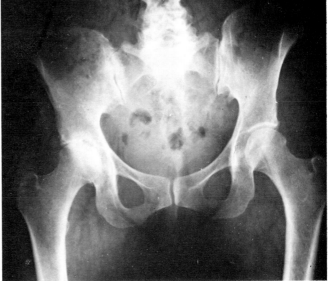

54

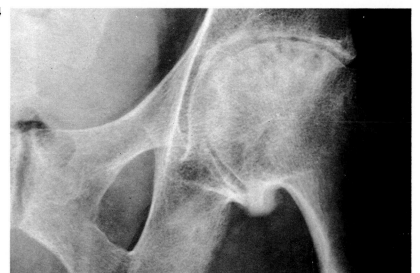

54 Moderate hip involvement in RA. In this close-up view, loss of cartilage from the whole femoral head is seen and there are erosions in its upper pole. Despite the osteophyte on the lower margin of the femoral head, there is minimal bony sclerosis. Once hip involvement is radiologically apparent, the outlook is poor. Total hip replacement should not be left too late, even in young patients, as continued weight-bearing may lead to acetabular deformity and protrusion of the joint into the pelvis, thus rendering surgery technically more difficult.

55

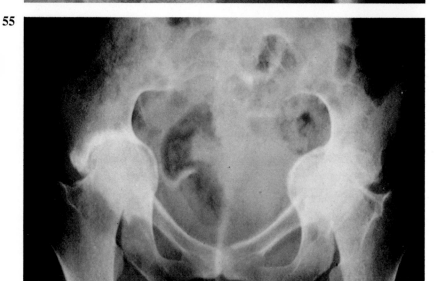

55 End-stage hip disease in RA. As with any inflammatory arthritis, the hip joint may migrate medially into the pelvis, producing the radiological appearances of protrusio acetabuli. This patient experienced severe restriction of all hip movements. Total hip replacement in a patient with protrusio acetabuli also necessitates reconstruction of the acetabulum and is best performed by a surgeon with a specific interest in RA.

56

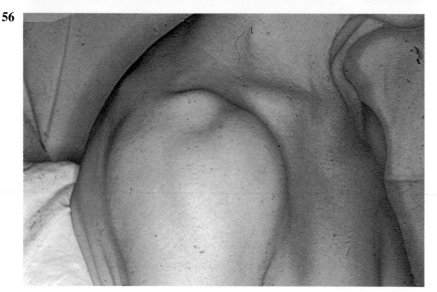

56 RA of the shoulder joint. Shoulder involvement is common in RA and may be the presenting complaint. Initially, a typical history of a painful arc of movement (*see* **328–335**) reflects rheumatoid synovitis of the subacromial bursa. This responds well to a local corticosteroid injection. Later, the joint itself is involved and more global restriction of joint movement develops. An effusion usually bulges anteriorly, as here. At this stage no radiological changes may be apparent, despite severely restricted movement.

57 Severe RA of the shoulder. One of the main functions of the rotator cuff muscles is to hold the head of the humerus down, allowing it to glide under the acromion and coracoacromial ligament during abduction. In RA, a tear in the rotator cuff occurs when synovitis in the subacromial bursa and/or the shoulder joint causes attenuation of the tendons. The tear then allows upward movement of the humeral head, as shown on this X-ray. Abduction and elevation of the shoulder are blocked as the deltoid pulls the head of the humerus directly against the acromium. Surgical repair of the rotator cuff is rarely successful in RA. Gross destruction of the head of the humerus is also seen on this film.

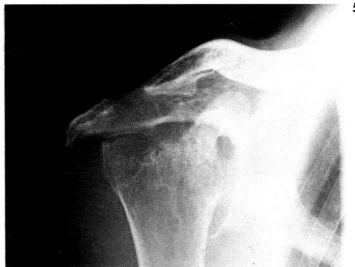

58 Late RA of the shoulder. The combination of a torn rotator cuff and severe destruction of the humeral head and the glenoid is often painful and very disabling. Shoulder replacement can be considered for severe pain, but it is technically unsatisfactory in all but a few hands, and rarely improves the existing range of movement. Here, the acromioclavicular joint is also severely eroded.

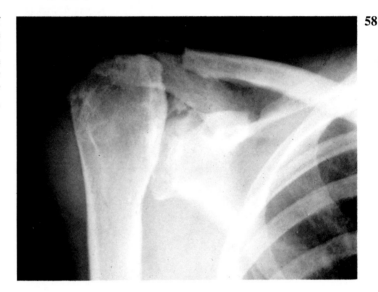

59 Olecranon bursitis. RA may cause massive olecranon bursitis, often with nodules in the bursa. Aspiration and injection with corticosteroid are helpful. However, the bursa may occasionally be infected; if infection is suspected, once the fluid has been aspirated and cultured, the patient will require antibiotics. In potentially infected cases a local corticosteroid injection should not be given (*see* pp.145–146).

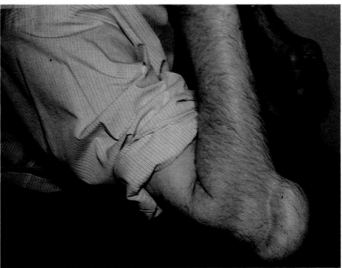

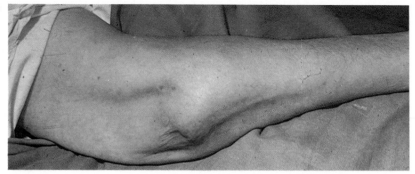

60 Involvement of the elbow in RA. Elbow synovitis and an effusion lead to painful extension and a fixed flexion deformity, making load carrying awkward. On examination, the effusion can be palpated, bulging into the space between the olecranon and the lateral epicondyle, as the elbow reaches the end of its range of extension. Pronation and supination may also become restricted due to involvement of the radial head. (These latter movements can also be restricted by wrist involvement, however.) If the pain and tenderness are mainly restricted to the radial head, where crepitus may be felt on rotation of the forearm, a local injection of the radiohumeral joint may be helpful. Surgical excision of the radial head is worthwhile when pain is persistent and severe.

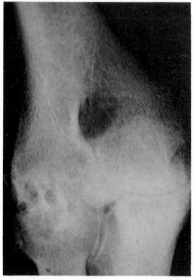

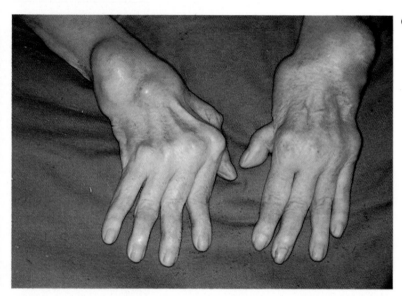

61 Advanced elbow involvement. There is complete destruction of the cartilage, with erosion of the radial head and of the lateral humeral epicondyle. The humeroulnar joint is also affected. Giant rheumatoid cysts, seen here in the humerus, may develop in any joint, but are most common around the elbow. Total elbow replacement is technically feasible in expert hands, although it is of more help in relieving pain than in restoring the range of movement.

62 Advanced wrist and hand involvement in RA – some typical deformities. This patient illustrates the devasting effects that long-standing RA can have on the hand. The deformities may coexist, as here, or appear independently. There is severe wasting of the dorsal interosseus muscles, and the fingers show volar subluxation of the MCP joints, combined with ulnar drift. The dominant right hand is typically worse

affected. All the fingers demonstrate fixed hyperextension of the PIP joints, combined with fixed flexion of the DIP joints. This combination is called a 'swan neck' deformity. Initially, such swan neck deformities may be reversible, and finger flexion remains possible. Frequently, however, flexion is lost and hand function becomes seriously impaired. Expert surgery may delay loss of function in reversible cases but, by the stage shown here, it is rarely effective. Various gadgets are available to help maintain the patient's independence (*see* Chapter 12).

This patient also has a 'Z-shaped' deformity of the right thumb, with fixed flexion of the MCP joint and hyperextension of the interphalangeal (IP) joint. This is caused by volar displacement of the thumb extensor tendons at the damaged first MCP joint.

The wrists are damaged, with florid synovitis and marked subluxation; early in the course of the disease the ulnar styloid may move dorsally, and this may be followed by palmar subluxation of the carpus on the forearm (as seen here in the left hand). Ulnar styloidectomy may help if pain is mainly restricted to the ulnar side. If pain is severe and movement restricted, the best solution is to fuse the wrist in slight dorsiflexion, a position which may produce some improvement in finger function (*see* p.161). Wrist splints are of use in some cases.

63 Advanced wrist and hand involvement in RA. Severe destruction and osteoporosis are seen both in the wrists and in the MCP joints (compare **17, 18 & 25–27**).

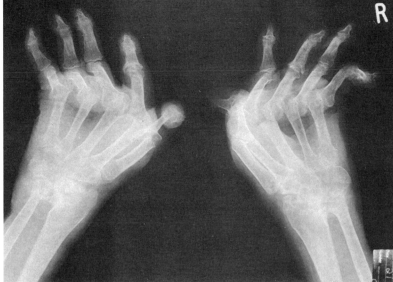

64 & 65 Infective arthritis in RA. Joints affected by RA are particularly susceptible to secondary infection, usually by blood-borne spread from an infected skin lesion such as an ulcerated metatarsal callosity (*see* **35**). Staphylococci are the most commonly isolated organisms. Unless the possibility of infection is borne constantly in mind, it is all too easy to assume that a sudden exacerbation of pain and swelling in a single or multiple joints is due to a flare of the disease. In this patient the wrist and elbow were secondarily infected via a foot ulcer; cellulitis made the infective nature of the flare clear.

Suspicion of joint infection constitutes a medical emergency and the patient will need urgent specialist referral. Antibiotics should not be prescribed before cultures of joint fluid, blood, urine and any other potentially infected site have been taken. Antibiotics may then be started immediately on the basis of a gram stain. If the patient is very ill, antibiotic treatment may be initiated 'blind', and adjusted later, once an infecting organism has been cultured and sensitivities obtained. In the absence of a positive culture, the best initial combination is either fucidic

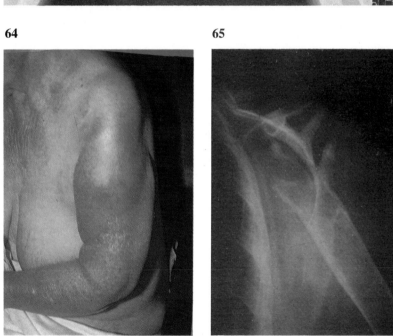

acid and flucloxacillin, or, assuming renal function is normal, fucidic acid and gentamicin (blood gentamicin levels are obligatory). Antibiotics should be given systemically for several days and continued orally for 8–12 weeks.

Early recognition of a pyoarthritis may prevent otherwise devastating joint destruction, such as that illustrated in this patient who had had a pyoarthritis of the shoulder (**65**).

66

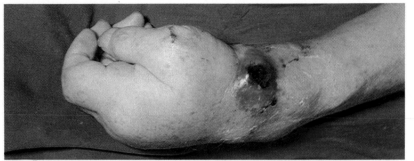

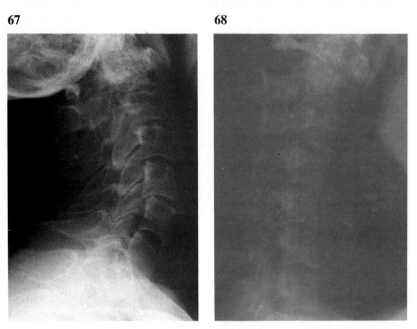

67 Cervical spine. The cervical spine is the only part of the axial skeleton to be significantly affected by rheumatoid arthritis. Synovitis occurs in the bursae that separate the odontoid process from its retaining structures, but its origin in the upper and midcervical vertebrae is unclear. Some doubt the presence of synovial neurocentral joints; others suggest that they are the site of synovitis. In this X-ray, taken with the neck held in extension, there is narrowing of the intervertebral disc between the third and fourth cervical vertebrae (C3/4) (in contrast to typical cervical spondylosis, where lower disc involvement is usual, *see* **160 & 161**), without reactive sclerosis or osteophyte formation, again in contrast with spondylosis. There is also slight backward movement (spondylolisthesis) of the body of C3 on C4 at this level. Such patients may develop nerve root entrapment at the affected cervical level, resulting in pain, paraesthesia, and loss of power and reflexes in a distribution determined by the nerve root affected. In this view the atlantoaxial region appears normal, although the odontoid is indistinct , suggesting that it is eroded.

68 Flexed cervical spine. When the patient is X-rayed with the neck in flexion, obvious involvement of the atlantoaxial joint may be demonstrated. In this case, there has been forward movement of the body of C1, due to damage to the retaining ligament by synovitis in the bursae that lie around the odontoid process. The distance from the anterior surface of the odontoid to the posterior arch of C2 measures 8 mm (normally less than 2–3 mm in flexion). A second film, with the neck in extension, will demonstrate whether the displacement is fixed or unstable. The X-ray finding of atlantoaxial instability may be asymptomatic or associated with severe pain, usually radiating to the occiput. Subluxation of the cervical spine at any level indicates that the patient is at risk of developing spinal cord compression. This is unpredictable, however, and may occur suddenly or insidiously, after many years of instability.

66 Pyoarthritis of the wrist. Clear signs of joint infection may be muted, especially in patients on long-term corticosteroids, and in the elderly and infirm. Other indicators, including fever, malaise and a potential source for the bacteraemia, should be sought. This elderly patient, on long-term corticosteroids for severe RA, had presented a few weeks previously with an infected penetrating ulcer on the foot. She subsequently became confused and unwell. Septicaemia was diagnosed when the wrist discharged pus.

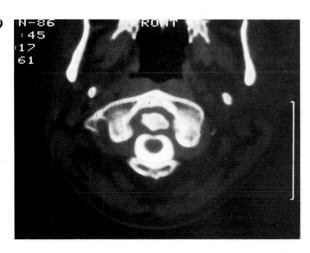

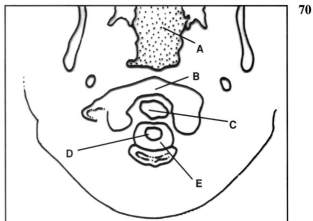

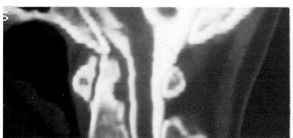

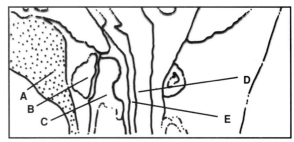

69–72 Cervical spine. MRI is a noninvasive technique, capable of visualising neck abnormalities in RA. In these T1-weighted films, erosions of the odontoid can be clearly seen in both the transverse (**69**) and the sagittal (**71**) views. The relationship of the odontoid to the cord is visible and normal: the cerebrospinal fluid (CSF) appears white, and the cord grey.

73 **74**

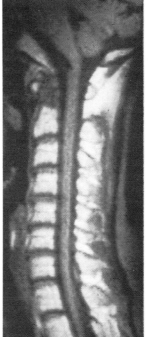

A = nasopharynx, B = anterior arch of atlas, C = odontoid process, D = spinal cord, E = cerebrospinal fluid.

73 & 74 Cervical spine. This T2-weighted scan shows the whole cervical spine, with the normal relationship of an eroded odontoid process which here lacks marrow and does not show up white like the rest of the vertebrae. The medulla and cerebellum are clearly seen. In T2-weighted films the CSF appears black and the cord grey. Hypertrophic chronic inflammatory synovial tissue arising from the bursa, which lies between the odontoid and its retaining transverse ligament, is detectable on a T2 scan; a soft tissue mass of this nature may contribute significantly to spinal cord compression. By taking films in flexion and extension, any spinal or medullary impingement may be seen.

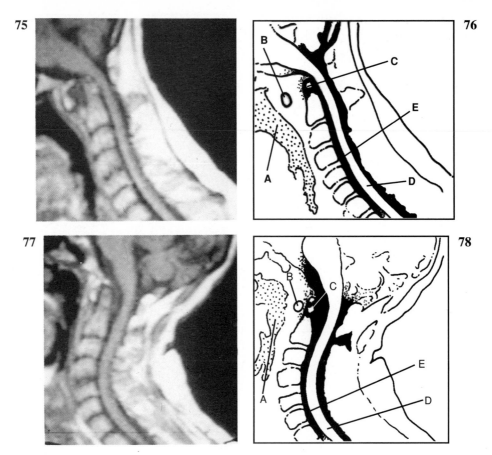

75–78 Cervical spine. In these T2-weighted MRI scans the odontoid is eroded and unstable. In the flexed view (**75 & 76**), there is obvious movement of the odontoid in relation to the anterior arch of the atlas. The already attenuated cord is angulated at this level by the displaced odontoid process. This pattern of subluxation at the atlantoaxial level can produce a spastic paraparesis, which may develop slowly and be difficult to detect because of the patient's generally impaired mobility and joint deformity. In **77 & 78** the spine is extended, the atlantoaxial distance reduced and the cord no longer impinged upon.

If any patient with RA describes increased difficulty in walking, without any obvious new articular cause, cervical myelopathy should be suspected.

In the near future it may be possible to use special flash sequences to produce cine MRI views of the unstable cervical spine during flexion and extension. CT myelography is another accurate method for demonstrating these changes, but it is an invasive procedure and should only be undertaken when surgery is being considered. Surgical correction may entail removal of the odontoid process and any abnormal synovium by a transoral approach, followed by a posterior fusion. This is a major, but potentially life-saving, procedure.

Although unpredictable, those at greatest risk of developing neurological complications from cervical spine involvement are patients, often male, with severe, remorselessly progressive, erosive, strongly seropositive, nodular disease. Long-term corticosteroid intake also appears to increase the risk.

(A = nasopharynx, B = anterior arch of atlas, C = odontoid process, D = spinal cord, E = cerebrospinal fluid.)

79 & 80 Cervical spine. Marked subluxation of C4 on C5, together with obliteration of the C5/6 disc space, can be seen on the plain film (**79**). The patient presented with a mixture of lower motor neuron symptoms and signs in the arms (weakness and paraesthesia), and a spastic paraparesis. The myelogram (**80**) shows a block at C4. Surgery was undertaken, but it was only partly effective and the patient remained chairbound.

Multilevel 'staircase' cervical subluxation may occur. Clinical signs in the arms are often helpful in localising the level to which surgery should be directed.

Any patient with known atlantoaxial subluxation or midcervical instability should be advised to inform physiotherapists, osteopaths, dentists and anaesthetists. Such patients are at risk of spinal cord damage by any manoeuvre that inadvertently causes sudden neck movements or requires the neck to be held in an awkward position for prolonged periods.

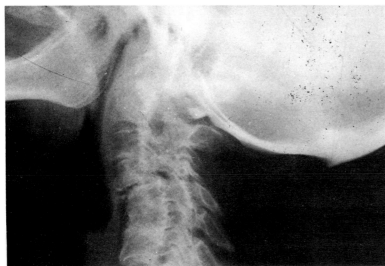

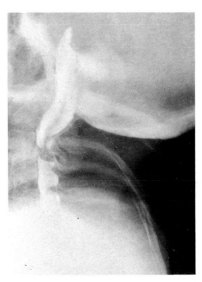

Extra-articular involvement

Cutaneous manifestations

Ulceration of the skin from a variety of causes is seen in RA. The ever-present risk that secondary infection may lead to bacteraemia and joint infection means that every attempt should be made to keep the lesion clean and to achieve healing. Avoidance of ill-fitting footwear and management of pressure points on the feet by appropriate chiropody or surgery are essential. With chair- or bed-bound patients the use of weight-distributing cushions, special mattresses and careful attention to regular turning to avoid pressure sores are vital. Special nursing care of bed-bound patients is essential as severe joint disease limits the individual's ability to move unaided.

81 Foot ulceration in RA. Deep ulceration may occur over subluxed metatarsal heads (*see* **35**) or, as here, over a rheumatoid nodule. The cause is increased local pressure and relative ischaemia. Alterations in footwear and the provision of moulded insoles to redistribute weight more evenly are helpful, but surgical forefoot arthroplasty may be necessary to prevent recurrence of ulceration over the metatarsal heads.

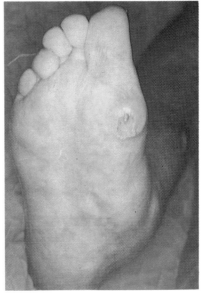

81

82

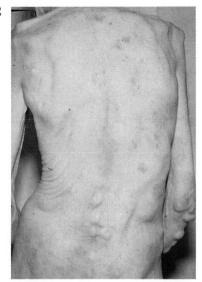

82 Ulcerated rheumatoid nodules. Multiple nodules may form in bed-bound patients. Without regular turning, the patient may develop secondary pressure ulceration, especially over the elbows, sacrum and sometimes the occiput. There is no alternative to careful nursing and the use of a low-air-loss or other special weight-distributing beds. A plastic surgeon should be consulted about excision of the nodules, and skin grafting should be performed if healing is delayed. Second-line drugs, aimed at controlling the disease process, may produce regression of the nodules.

83

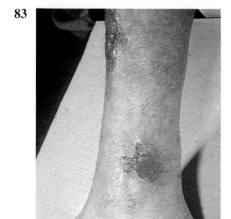

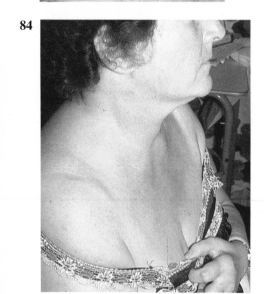

83 Ulceration of the lower leg. Leg ulceration is relatively common in RA and has a variety of causes. The skin becomes thin and atrophic and is easily damaged, especially if the patient is on corticosteroids. There may be a degree of venous stasis due to reduced mobility and impairment of the muscular venous pump. In patients with active arthritis, there may be an underlying vasculitis. Vasculitic ulcers can be very painful and difficult to treat. Occasionally, they warrant admission to hospital.

84 & 85 Drug eruption. Generalised skin rashes are not a common feature of adult RA, but may be due to unrelated factors or a drug reaction. A variety of cutaneous responses occurs with anti-inflammatory and second-line drugs. Some patients experience photosensitivity (**84**), with the rash confined to light-exposed areas (e.g. with fenbufen or sulphasalazine), while local patches of dermatitis or a more generalised eruption may occur in others, as in the patient in **85**, who was receiving gold therapy. Withdrawal of the drug is usually obligatory. Short-term use of local corticosteroid creams may be necessary and occasionally, in the rare, exfoliative reaction, oral corticosteroids are required.

84

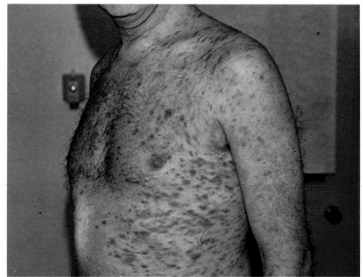

85

86 Nail fold vasculitis. Patients with sero-positive RA may develop crops of small, initially painful, brownish red lesions around the cuticle or nail fold. The pathology is an underlying endarteritis due to immune-complex deposition, with secondary local thrombosis. The lesions usually occur during active phases of the disease and may indicate the need for an immunosuppressive agent such as azathioprine or methotrexate.

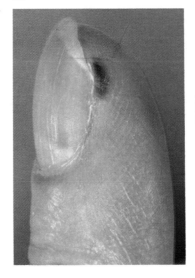

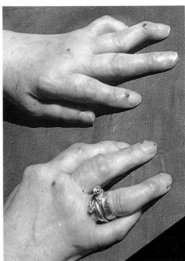

87 Small artery vasculitis. In some patients, nail fold vasculitis is part of a more widespread condition involving larger vessels, in which case cutaneous lesions develop more extensively. If such patients are smokers, they should be strongly advised to stop.

Cardiovascular system manifestations

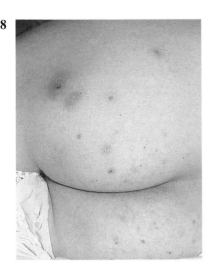

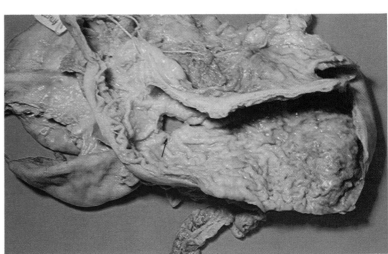

88 Small vessel vasculitis. A spectrum of vasculitic lesions is found in RA, some of which are subclinical and found only at *postmortem* examination. Capillaritis and venulitis underlie rheumatoid synovitis and the formation of rheumatoid nodules. Necrotising arteritis may present as benign but painful cutaneous lesions, as seen in this patient, but it may also have a more explosive onset with fever and a polymorphonuclear leucocytosis. At times, it is indistinguishable from polyarteritis nodosa, both clinically and pathologically (*see* p.108). Pathologically, there is intimal hypertrophy and a variable degree of arterial wall and perivascular inflammation. In milder cases, there is neither medial involvement nor damage to the internal elastic lamina.

89 Obliterative arteritis. This type of arterial damage is thought to be caused by immune-complex deposition. Patients are usually strongly seropositive for rheumatoid factors and may have circulating immune complexes in the serum, and serological evidence of complement activation. Immuno-histochemical staining of the vessels reveals IgM, IgG and complement products deposited in the vessel walls. Although the most common cause of acute abdominal pain in RA is peptic ulceration due to drugs, very acute pain may be due to an arteritis involving the blood supply to the gut causing perforation (here of the stomach) or gangrene. These are usually seen in patients with fulminating arteritis and are among the rare causes of death in RA.

90

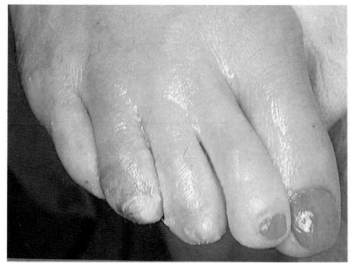

90 Digital gangrene. Larger vessel arteritis is rare and a poor prognostic indicator, suggesting multisystem involvement. Arteriography may aid the detection of any coincidental but treatable localised atheromatous lesion. Otherwise, vasodilators and/or high dose intravenous boluses of methylprednisolone or cyclophosphamide may be needed. There is a significant mortality in such patients, due to myocardial ischaemia, cerebrovascular accidents or multiple perforations of the gut. Peripheral neuropathies may also be caused by arteritis (*see* **108**).

91

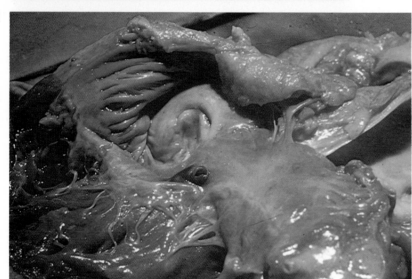

91 Cardiac lesions in RA. Although the heart can be affected in a variety of ways in RA, significant clinical disease is uncommon and it is frequently only demonstrable at *postmortem* examination. Pericarditis may occur, and rheumatoid nodules may form in the pericardium, myocardium or valves, causing conduction defects or, rarely, valvular insufficiency. Myocardial infarction may develop due to a coronary arteritis. Illustrated here is the heart of a patient who died suddenly due to rupture of the sinus of Valsalva, at the site of a myocardial rheumatoid nodule.

Pleuropulmonary manifestations

Most respiratory symptoms that occur in patients with RA are due to common and coincidental disorders. Bronchiectasis and chronic bronchitis associated with RA may reflect abnormalities of the respiratory mucosa due to Sjögren's syndrome (*see* **98–100**). Some respiratory manifestations, however, are directly related to the disease process.

92 & 93 Solitary rheumatoid lung nodule. Single or multiple opacities in the periphery of the lungs may be asymptomatic. They occur most commonly in male patients who have multiple subcutaneous rheumatoid nodules elsewhere. If present on the pleural surface, they may produce a reactive effusion (*see* **94**). Complications include cavitation, visible tomographically (**93**) or by CT scan. The cavity may become secondarily infected or, rarely, may rupture into the pleural cavity, causing a pneumothorax or pyopneumothorax. Histologically, the lesions resemble typical rheumatoid nodules (*see* **12**). A biopsy may be necessary to exclude a coincidental primary or secondary malignant deposit.

92

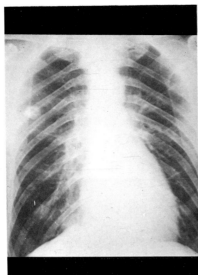

93

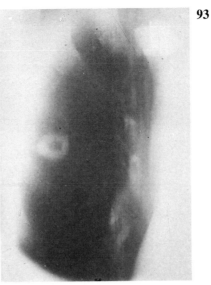

94

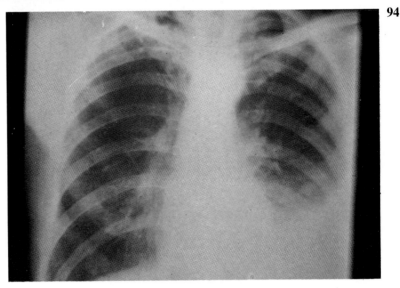

94 Rheumatoid pleural effusion. Pleural involvement may be unilateral or bilateral, and is usually asymptomatic, often resolving spontaneously or as the arthritis remits. Pleuritic pain may occur and a large effusion causes shortness of breath. A diagnostic pleural tap reveals opalescent rather than purulent fluid, with the features of an exudate. Microscopically, there is usually a lot of amorphous debris and a variable number of polymorphs and/or monocytic cells. It may be difficult to distinguish from an infectious cause, so the fluid should be cultured. Interestingly, the glucose level is usually low, even in noninfected RA pleural effusions. A positive rheumatoid factor test in the fluid may be helpful but is not diagnostic.

95

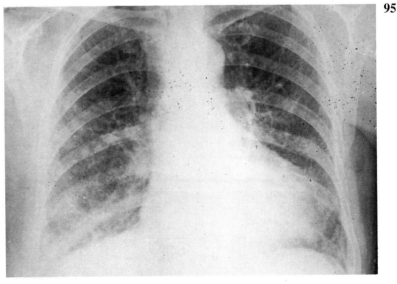

95 Interstitial lung disease. Interstitial fibrosing alveolitis, indistinguishable from the idiopathic variety, may occur in RA. Typically, patients present with progressive shortness of breath, a nonproductive cough and fixed crepitations in the basal zones on auscultation. Initially, chest X-rays reveal diffuse basal interstitial fibrosis with a mottled pattern. Here, the honeycomb appearance of more established disease is seen clearly in the patient's right base, and there are early changes in the upper zones. Pulmonary function tests demonstrate a restrictive ventilatory pattern, with reduced compliance and impaired gas transfer.

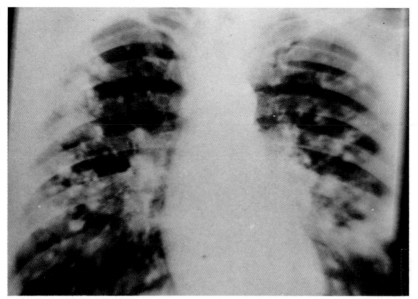

96 Caplan's syndrome. RA patients who have a history of dust exposure (coal miners, asbestos workers and chalk miners) may develop a very striking form of lung disease. Multiple, well-defined and mainly peripheral lung nodules are seen on X-ray, superimposed on a background picture of pneumoconiosis. Smaller nodules may coalesce or cavitate. These lung changes may predate the development of clinical joint involvement. In many countries this is a notifiable occupational disease, and affected patients may be eligible for compensation.

Ocular manifestations and Sjögren's syndrome

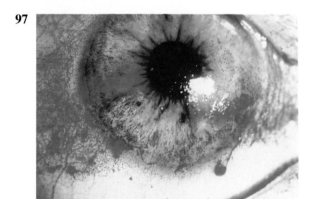

97 Keratoconjunctivitis sicca. Dry eyes that cause gritty discomfort are common in RA, and may be associated with dryness of the mouth and reduced respiratory mucosal secretions – the sicca syndrome. The eye is slightly reddened and there is reduced tear secretion, measurable with a Schirmer's test: a standard, sterile piece of blotting paper is hooked over the lower lid for 5 minutes, with the eye closed. Tear secretion is measured in terms of the length of moistened paper: less than 5 mm is diagnostic and 5–10 mm is suspicious.

The results of the sicca syndrome can be clearly demonstrated by applying a small amount of Rose Bengal stain to the eye (a painful test which should not be performed routinely). Patchy pink staining of the cornea and scleral conjunctiva indicates superficial erosions. Attached filaments of corneal epithelium are also visible here. Regular use of artificial tears (hypromellose drops) reduces the symptoms.

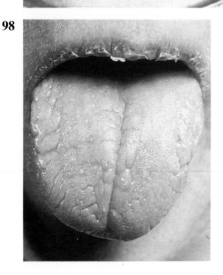

98 Sjögren's syndrome. This disorder is most commonly seen in patients with seropositive RA, but it may also occur in other connective tissue diseases, such as systemic lupus erythematosus or progressive systemic sclerosis (*see* p.108). A primary form, in which patients have no associated autoimmune disorder, also exists. The sicca complex is associated with diffuse infiltration of the exocrine glands by lymphocytes and plasma cells, and with painless enlargement of the parotid glands. Most patients are female and present with oral and ocular dryness and occasional painful parotitis. In extreme cases the dryness is so acute that swallowing and speech are affected. In general, treatment is symptomatic, but in severe cases corticosteroids or cyclophosphamide may be considered.

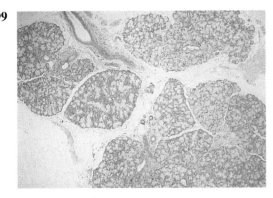

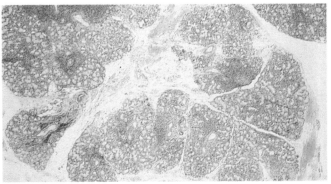

99 & 100 Labial gland biopsy in Sjögren's syndrome. Histopathology can be obtained by a simple labial gland biopsy. When compared with the normal appearance (**99**), the Sjögren's biopsy (**100**) shows marked infiltration by lymphocytes and plasma cells, with areas of acinar tissue replaced by lymphocytic foci. Minor changes may be difficult to distinguish from those of normal aging in elderly patients, but are diagnostic in those under 50 years of age.

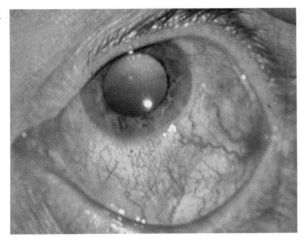

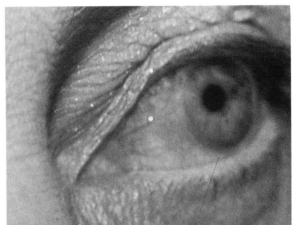

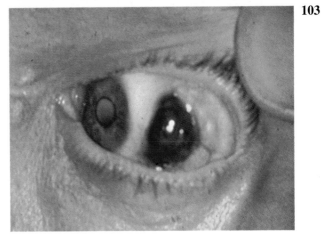

101 Rheumatoid episcleritis. Generally a self-limiting condition that gives rise to mild ocular discomfort but no visual abnormality, rheumatoid episcleritis is due to inflammation of the superficial layers of the sclera and causes a raised inflamed area surrounded by intense injection of the superficial conjunctival vessels. It generally resolves in a few weeks and requires no treatment.

102 Rheumatoid scleritis. Rheumatoid scleritis is more painful and potentially more serious than episcleritis. It is often bilateral and usually occurs in severe seropositive disease. A raised, yellowish red lesion, often in the superior sclera, is associated with localised hyperaemia of the deep scleral vessels giving a more diffuse redness than that seen in episcleritis. Although it may resolve, the condition is frequently recurrent and patients should be referred urgently for specialist advice. Local corticosteroid drops are used if the pain is severe. Rarely, the choroid and ciliary body may also be affected.

103 Scleromalacia perforans. Severe scleritis may lead to permanent localised thinning of the sclera, which develops a bluish tinge. The sclera may subsequently perforate, a complication resulting in blindness.

104

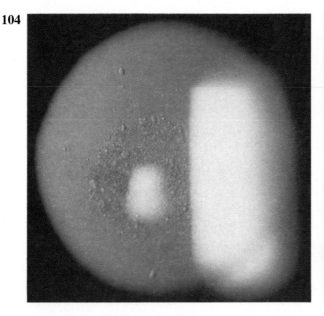 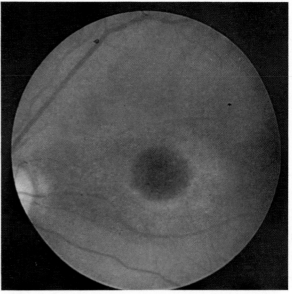

104 Cataract. Posterior subcapsular cataracts are a relatively common complication of long-term corticosteroid therapy, although such therapy is now less frequently used in RA than previously. Initially, the patient complains of blurred vision and of halos around bright lights. As the cataract develops, vision deteriorates and surgical cataract extraction may be necessary. The changes in the lens are best seen by slit-lamp examination (as here), but are often visible by simple ophthalmoscopy.

105 Retinal damage due to chloroquine. High doses of chloroquine, given over prolonged periods for RA, have caused damage to the fovea and permanent central visual loss in this patient. Such a serious complication is unlikely to occur with the low doses of hydroxychloroquine, used over shorter periods, which are more usual today. Nonetheless, most rheumatologists recommend ocular checks, including visual field measurements, before and at regular intervals during treatment with chloroquine or hydroxychloroquine.

Neurological manifestations

The most common neurological complications of RA are nerve entrapments in the carpal tunnel or, less commonly, in the tarsal tunnel. The latter produces numbness and paraesthesia over the heel, sole and medial aspect of the foot. Entrapment of the ulnar nerve may occur at the elbow, or of cervical roots as they emerge from the spine (*see* **67 & 68**) A variety of presentations of peripheral neuropathy may be seen, but the central nervous system (CNS) is generally spared.

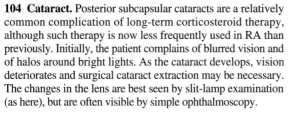

106 & 107 Carpal tunnel syndrome. Carpal tunnel syndrome presents with a history of painful paraesthesia and numbness in a median nerve distribution –index finger, thumb, middle and ring fingers. However, it is not uncommon for only part of this distribution to be affected. The symptoms are typically worse in the early hours of the morning and may waken the patient. The simplest treatment is to provide a resting splint to wear at night for a few weeks (**107**). This may relieve the symptoms permanently or temporarily; even temporary benefit is diagnostic, however, establishing that the symptoms are not arising from the neck. If splinting fails, a local injection (*see* **339 & 340**) or surgical decompression of the inflamed tendon sheaths in the carpal tunnel should be considered. If there is diagnostic doubt, nerve conduction studies should be performed to demonstrate a lesion in the carpal tunnel. Slowing of conduction at the wrist may be found and, in more severe cases, fasciculation potentials in the thenar muscles.

In severe cases, where there is already established thenar muscle wasting (see the right hand) or permanent numbness, the patient should be referred urgently for nerve conduction studies and surgical decompression, without a prior injection.

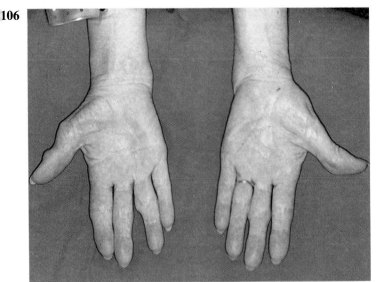

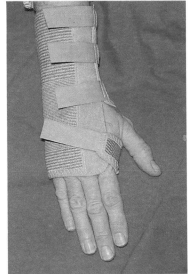

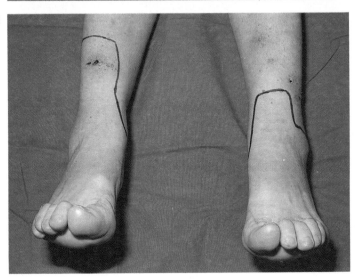

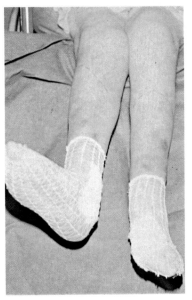

108 Bilateral peripheral sensory neuropathy. This patient had a symmetrical peripheral neuropathy with numbness and paraesthesia. Vasculitis of the vasa nervorum was confirmed on sural nerve biopsy. Vasculitic leg ulcers are also visible. Although extensive vasculitis may have a poor prognosis, this patient remained alive 6 years after the film was taken, with little evidence of extension of the neuropathy.

109 Mononeuritis multiplex. Vasculitis may also produce a patchy sensory loss and foot or wrist drop, due to mononeuritis multiplex. The foot (or wrist) should be supported in a splint. Corticosteroids may help, but recovery is often incomplete.

Renal manifestations and other rarer complications of RA

RA rarely affects the kidneys directly. Proteinuria and/or haematuria are most commonly due to an intercurrent infection or to side-effects of drugs such as gold or D-penicillamine. Analgesic nephropathy or interstitial nephritis due to nonsteroidal anti-inflammatory drugs (NSAIDs) may also occur. Persistent haematuria without proteinuria warrants investigation to rule out renal tract malignancy.

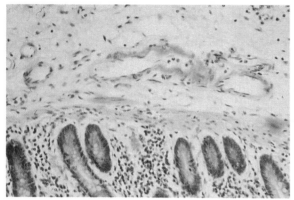

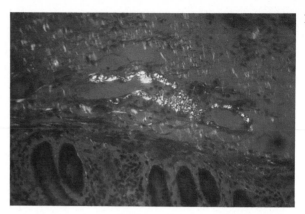

110 & 111 Rectal biopsy of amyloid disease in RA. In long-standing RA, reactive secondary amyloidosis (formerly 'secondary'), also known as AA-type amyloidosis, may occur. The precursor protein is a circulating acute-phase reactant called serum amyloid A (SAA) protein. This type of amyloidosis generally presents as proteinuria or the nephrotic syndrome and may cause death due to chronic renal failure.

Investigations should include measurement of the glomerular filtration rate (GFR) and of 24-hour urine protein excretion. Amyloid can be detected in most affected patients by performing a full-thickness rectal biopsy. On a haematoxylin and eosin stain amyloid appears as amorphous pink deposits, predominantly around blood vessels of the submucosa. Amyloid protein also binds to the dye Congo Red, staining an orange-red (**110**). When such a preparation is examined under polarised light, it manifests a characteristic apple-green or yellow-green birefringence, known as dichroism (**111**) (*see also* **315** and p.143).

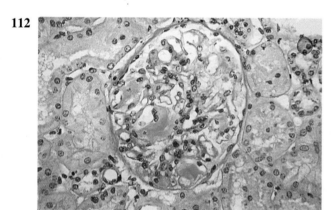

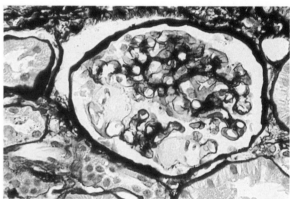

112 & 113 Amyloid deposits in the kidney. A renal biopsy may be needed to confirm the presence of amyloid, or to exclude other renal lesions. The glomerular capillary walls are thickened by amyloid deposition, which is amorphous and here stains pink with periodic acid Schiff stain (**112**), but does not take up silver stain (**113**). Chlorambucil and other cytotoxic agents may slow the development of renal failure due to amyloidosis, but the outlook remains poor and mortality is high. New scanning techniques make it possible to visualise amyloid deposits *in vivo*, improving the assessment of this potentially fatal disease and offering hope in its treatment.

114 Lymphoedema, lymphadenopathy and Felty's syndrome. Localised or generalised painless lymphadenopathy occurs in RA, affecting nodes proximal to inflamed joints. If the nodes are tender, an infective arthritis should be ruled out. Occasionally, lymphoedema of the arm arises (here affecting the right arm), probably reflecting lymphatic dysfunction.

Sometimes, splenomegaly and neutropenia, collectively known as **Felty's syndrome**, are seen in RA patients. In such

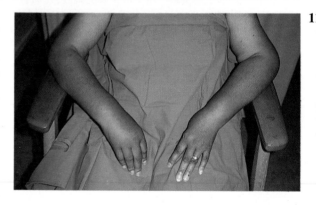

patients, leg ulceration and recurrent infections may occur. In some cases splenectomy is helpful; in others cautious treatment with cytotoxic agents is advocated.

Treatment of RA

Early disease

Achieving a balance between comforting reassurance and a realistic appraisal of the short- and long-term outlook is difficult but important. Although anxiety about the future is understandable, it is often worse than necessary as, once the initial flare has settled, function improves significantly, even if gradual deterioration may again occur in the longer term. It is important to involve patient's partners in early consultations so that they understand and share in the process. In some cases, formal counselling may be helpful to reduce anxiety levels and to enable the development of better coping strategies. General advice about rest must be realistic in young and busy people, but it is often possible for them to pace their lives better or to ask the help of friends and relatives. A physiotherapist will be able to teach a simple series of exercises to maintain fitness and joint movements, and an occupational therapist can advise about resting splints and basic modifications of daily activities.

During the early stages of the disease, symptomatic treatment with a combination of simple analgesics and NSAIDs is appropriate. Provided that upper dose limits are clearly stated, patients may be left to decide whether or not to take them, according to the severity of their symptoms. The more common potential side-effects should be discussed, and the patient told what to do if they occur. The use of nocturnal slow-release preparations or suppositories of NSAIDs helps to control the early morning pain and stiffness that are so typical of this and of other inflammatory arthritides. A hot bath or shower in the morning is also helpful.

Many patients are keen to try complementary measures, such as dietary changes, herbal remedies, acupuncture or homoeopathy. With the possible exception of diet, there is little evidence that such treatments offer any significant long-term improvement, but many patients nonetheless appear to derive symptomatic benefit. In practical terms it is not important whether the effect is real or a placebo response, provided that individuals continue to take appropriate orthodox medications and are doing themselves no harm. Dietary manipulations, for example, excluding specific foods, or adopting an elemental diet and then gradually reintroducing food systematically to see if any produces a flare, do seem to help some individuals. If patients are keen to experiment, it is reasonable to encourage them, as long as they are carefully supervised to ensure that they maintain a good nutritional balance and do not cause too many difficulties for the rest of their family. Changing to a diet containing fewer saturated fatty acids, with fish oil or evening primrose oil supplements, is expensive, but it may reduce the need for NSAIDs, at least in mild cases. Such a diet appears to alter the normal metabolic pathways of prostaglandins and other inflammatory mediators, which are derived from precursor dietary fatty acids, towards different mediators that are less proinflammatory.

Progressive disease

A proportion of patients, perhaps 25%, go into spontaneous remission or achieve satisfactory control of symptoms and show no evidence of progressive joint damage. Others, despite reasonable symptomatic control, show evidence of continuing synovitis and joint damage, and require more aggressive treatment. The main second-line drugs available are enteric coated sulphasalazine, oral or intramuscular gold salts, D-penicillamine, azathioprine and weekly oral methotrexate (*see* **Table 3**). Although it is not claimed that such drugs cure RA, there is evidence that they retard its more serious and progressive effects, particularly when measured in terms of erosions on X-rays. Thus, they may decrease long-term disability. They are potentially toxic, but so too are NSAIDs, and careful monitoring has reduced the risk of severe and irreversible side-effects.

Not treating RA is also risky; the risk of doing nothing must be carefully weighed up against the risk of taking drugs. If active RA does not show signs of settling, many rheumatologists now treat relatively early disease (within the first 3–6 months) with enteric coated sulphasalazine. If this is not beneficial, or produces side-effects, other slightly more toxic drugs may be tried.

More controversially, combinations of these second-line agents are being employed in patients with more aggressive disease, but only under specialist supervision. Once-weekly methotrexate has produced dramatic benefits in severe disease and where other drugs have failed, but it is potentially toxic and again should only be used under close specialist supervision.

Once the decision has been made to recommend second-line agents, patients should be fully informed of the potential benefits and side-effects. The unpredictability of individual responses should also be discussed with patients and their primary health care team, together with the implications of starting second-line treatment in terms of a commitment to longer-term treatment and to regular monitoring to detect progressive damage, relapse and side-effects. Patients who are able to understand the importance of monitoring for side-effects should be given some responsibility for their own monitoring.

Corticosteroid drugs are mainly used as local intra-articular or soft tissue injections, and these are discussed elsewhere (Chapter 10). Occasional intramuscular depot injections or high-dose oral boluses are appropriate in acute generalised flares. The problem with longer-term corticosteroid therapy is that patients often lose the striking initial benefit and find it increasingly difficult to stop taking the drug without developing a flare. The long-term complications of steroids, particularly those of skin thinning and osteoporosis, may greatly complicate the later management of patients and increase their long-term disability .

Continuing attention to exercise and physiotherapy, with provision of splints and other aids, is essential. The close involvement of an orthopaedic surgeon with an interest in the surgical management of RA, preferably in a combined clinic with a rheumatologist, helps when considering early synovectomy of joints or tendon sheaths, and when planning reconstructive surgery.

Table 3. Dose ranges for second-line drugs in RA.

Hydroxychloroquine	**200 mg once or twice daily; reduce to 5 days per week when possible**
	Skin rashes
	Retinal damage – precludes long-term use; 6–8-monthly slit-lamp and visual field examination mandatory
Sulphasalazine EC	**500 mg, increasing to 2–3 g daily after food**
	Nausea (increase dose slowly)
	Skin rashes (desensitisation can be tried)
	Liver function disturbance
	Occasional thrombocytopenia or neutropenia
	Regular liver function tests and full blood counts mandatory
Sodium aurothiomalate	**Test dose 5–10 mg, then 20–50 mg weekly. Reduce frequency with improvement**
	Skin rashes and mouth ulcers
	Neutropenia or thrombocytopenia
	Renal changes
	Monthly full blood count and weekly urine testing mandatory
Auranofin	**3 mg daily, increasing to 6 mg daily**
	Diarrhoea – usually mild
	Skin rashes and mouth ulcers
	Neutropenia or thrombocytopenia
	Renal changes
	Monthly full blood count and weekly urine testing mandatory
D-penicillamine	**250 mg daily *before food*, increasing to 250 mg two or three times daily**
	Nausea
	Skin rashes
	Neutropenia or thrombocytopenia
	Renal changes
	Occasionally induces antinuclear antibodies
	Regular full blood count and urine testing mandatory
Azathioprine	**25 mg increasing to 50 mg twice a day – maximum 2.5 mg/kg/day**
	Nausea
	Neutropenia or thrombocytopenia
	Monthly full blood count and liver function tests mandatory
Methotrexate	**2.5 mg *weekly* increasing to 15-20 mg *weekly***
	Mouth ulcers, diarrhoea, nausea and vomiting – may be helped by giving 15 mg folinic (NOT folic) acid 18 hours after methotrexate
	Liver function changes
	Neutropenia and thrombocytopenia
	Rarely pulmonary fibrosis; routine lung function tests/chest X-ray indicated
	Monthly full blood count and liver function tests mandatory

3 Osteoarthritis

Osteoarthritis (OA) is the name applied to a common and, to some extent, age-related process that affects synovial joints. Some rheumatologists still prefer to use the term 'osteoarthrosis' in order to emphasise that inflammation, although present, appears to play a relatively unimportant role in the pathology. The alternative term of 'degenerative joint disease' is also used but is less acceptable to the patient.

The definition of OA is complex. There are typical histological changes which occur in the cartilage, subchondral and periarticular bone (*see* **118**) and, to a lesser extent, in the synovium. The radiological appearances are essential for diagnosis (**Table 4**), but their significance can only be determined in the context of the clinical symptoms and signs.

The clinical diagnosis of OA is confirmed by correlating the clinical picture with the typical radiological appearances. However, this process has its limitations because, with advancing age, there is an increase in the prevalence of such radiological changes in the population, but their relationship to symptoms is extremely variable. Ultimately, the diagnosis rests upon assessment of the relevance of the clinical and radiological findings to the presenting symptoms, and upon elimination of other possible causes of pain, such as local soft tissue lesions, pain referred from a more proximal site, coincidental inflammatory arthritis, or a more generalised cause of pain such as polymyalgia rheumatica (*see* p.135) or primary fibromyalgia (*see* p.155).

OA exists in both a primary form, which has a genetic determinant and is age-related to some extent, and a secondary form, in which the joint changes develop in a joint that has been previously damaged by a variety of predisposing causes, for example, trauma, previous irreversible joint damage due to arthritis, or certain congenital joint abnormalities (**Table 5**). Thus, a torn semilunar cartilage (meniscus) of the knee will often predispose to early OA, specifically in the affected compartment; this is independent of whether the damaged cartilage is excised or not. Certain sports appear to lead to the earlier development of OA, possibly only in those who already have a hereditary predisposition. Thus, football and basketball players develop OA of the knee, boxers develop OA of the MCP joints and ballet dancers develop OA of the ankle.

Table 4. Radiological features of OA (*see* **115**).

Reduction of joint space = cartilage thinning
Periarticular osteophyte formation
Subchondral bone sclerosis and cyst formation

Table 5. Classification of OA.

Primary	Nodal pattern – restricted to the hands	
	Generalised OA (with nodal OA of hands)	
	Hip OA	
Secondary	Congenital	Congenital dislocation of the hip
	Traumatic	Meniscal tear of the knee
		Fracture through a joint
	Inflammatory	Following previous inflammatory or septic arthritis
	Endocrine	Acromegaly
	Metabolic	Haemochromatosis
		Wilson's disease
Pseudo-OA	Calcium pyrophosphate deposition (*see* **156 & 157**)	

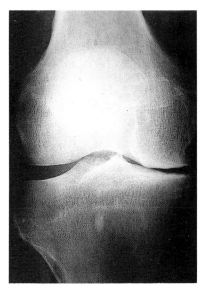

115

115 OA of the knee.

Pathology

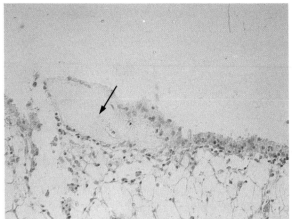

116 Cartilage shard in the synovium. Although synovial biopsies are becoming increasingly available from arthroscopic investigations, the changes seen in OA are nonspecific and provide variable evidence of inflammation. Appearances such as this, where a shard of separated cartilage (arrow) lies in the superficial synovium and is causing mild local inflammation, may support the view that the aetiology of OA is, in part, inflammatory.

The identification of a variety of crystals, including calcium hydroxyapatite and calcium orthophosphate, in osteoarthritic joints has led to increasing interest in the possibility of an inflammatory component to the disease. A particularly severe form of OA, with a different pattern of joint involvement, is occasionally associated with chondrocalcinosis – the deposition of calcium pyrophosphate crystals in hyaline and fibrous cartilage (*see* **156** & **157**).

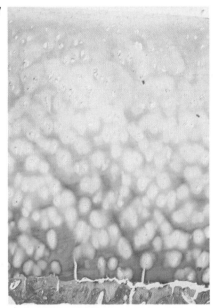

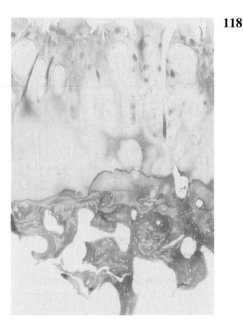

117 & 118 Histological appearances of OA. The earliest changes of OA appear in the cartilage. It is thought that biochemical abnormalities of the cartilage, involving its constituent collagen and proteoglycans, are the primary abnormality. These abnormalities lead to reduced hydration of the cartilage and alter its physical properties. The normal compressibility and resistance to shearing forces are lost, with surface fibrillation and fissuring leading to eventual degradation. The subarticular bone demonstrates a complex response, which produces sclerosis and remodelling abnormalities at the margins of the articular surface, resulting in the formation of periarticular osteophytes. This is not a simple degenerative process, but an active one. It presumably occurs as a result of reduced protection from the overlying, abnormal cartilage, and is perhaps also due to loss of normal local cytokine control by chondrocytes. The normal histology (stained with Masson's trichrome) is shown in **117**, while the abnormal section (**118**) reveals fibrillation of the surface cartilage, with deep fissuring of the cartilage and sclerosis of the subarticular bone.

Clinical manifestations

119 Nodal OA, demonstrating Heberden's nodes. The most common manifestation of OA in the hands is involvement of the distal interphalangeal joints. Initially, there may be pain, redness and swelling of the joint. This may superficially resemble and be confused with psoriatic arthritis (*see* **196**). The pain settles after a few weeks or months, leaving bony swellings called Heberden's nodes: these are the hallmark of nodal OA. They are more common in women than in men and there is usually a family history of similar hand involvement, although the severity varies from generation to generation. In a small proportion of patients, Heberden's nodes are associated with OA of other joints, particularly the knees. A more extensive, generalised OA can occur, but patients should be reassured that this is uncommon and that the risk is not great.

Occasionally, a painless cystic swelling develops. This may rupture, discharging clear, yellow, viscous jelly. Such swellings are not serious, should be kept dry and clean, and will usually settle. Surgical removal is rarely successful.

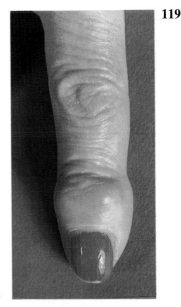

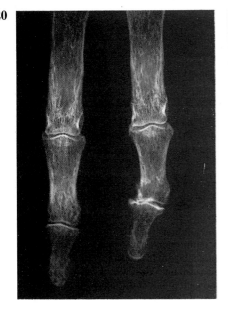

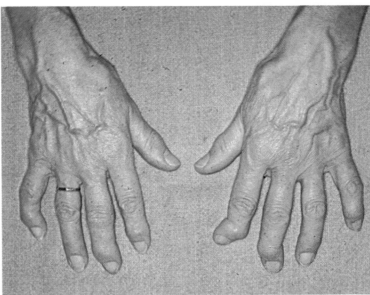

120 Heberden's node on X-ray. Initially, only soft tissue swelling is apparent radiologically. However, as the bony nodes form, so the typical appearances of OA become obvious with reduction of joint space (which reflects loss of cartilage thickness) and osteophyte formation. In addition to these features, this patient also demonstrates the deformity (here of the DIP joint of the index finger) that frequently develops. Subarticular bone cysts may also occur. Similar changes occur less frequently in the PIP joints (*see* **122** & **123**).

121 Advanced Heberden's nodes. With time, the generally painless bony swellings stabilise in size, although there may still be progressive change, with deviation of the distal phalanx, as seen here in the left index and both middle fingers. This is unsightly, but severe disability is uncommon. Surgery has no place in the management of DIP joint involvement. However, surgical stabilisation of an unstable thumb IP joint may improve hand function considerably.

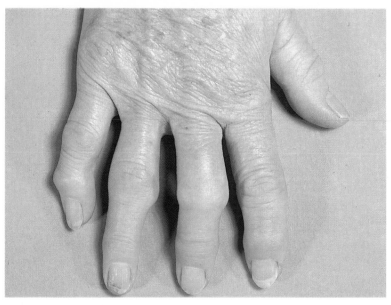

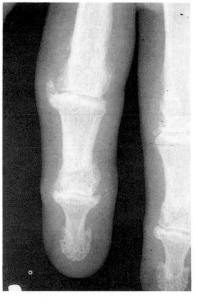

122 Bouchard's nodes. The bony swellings of nodal OA are called Bouchard's nodes when they affect the PIP joints. Although less commonly affected than the DIP joints, PIP joints follow the same clinical course. Resultant reduction of finger flexion may, however, cause more disability than with DIP involvement. There are often associated Heberden's nodes, but these may be minimal and such a picture can lead to confusion with RA. In OA the swelling is not associated with an inflammatory polyarthritis, however, and the subsequent development of bony nodes provides the diagnostic key.

123 Heberden's and Bouchard's nodes on X-ray. In this advanced case the cardinal radiological changes of OA can be seen, with loss of cartilage thickness, osteophyte formation and subchondral bone sclerosis of both the DIP and PIP joints.

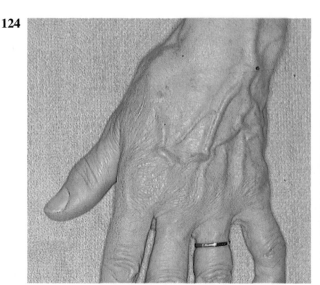

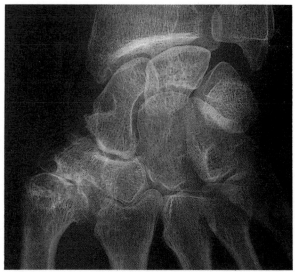

124 & 125 Osteoarthritis of the first carpometacarpal joint. The base of the thumb is often involved in nodal OA, causing localised pain, especially on squeezing or gripping, and tenderness. The pain generally settles spontaneously within a few months, but the joint becomes stiffened and adducted to produce the 'square' hand of OA. Local coarse crepitus can often be felt during movement, with osteophyte formation and loss of joint space visible on X-ray.

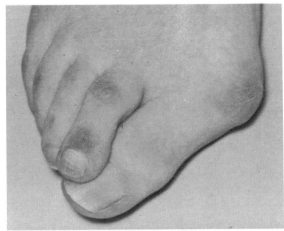

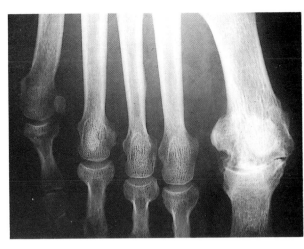

126 & 127 Hallux rigidus. The deformity of hallux valgus (**126**) is common and often asymptomatic, apart from the risk of developing a bunion overlying the first MTP joint due to pressure from shoes. Some patients also experience marked stiffening and crepitus of the first MTP joint (hallux rigidus), which limits walking and may occur with or without hallux valgus. Radiologically, there is florid osteophyte formation and loss of joint space. The use of a metatarsal rocker bar on the shoe to prevent dorsiflexion during walking may help, or surgery may occasionally be necessary.

128 Early OA of the knee. After the hand, the knee is the next most common joint to develop OA. Mild pain on weight-bearing, intermittent creaking on flexion, and a tendency to stiffen after inactivity are the presenting symptoms. Occasionally, an effusion, with resultant pain and stiffness, may occur. If one compartment is affected, the pain may be unilateral, occurring along the joint line. Local causes of pain, such as medial or lateral ligament strain, infrapatellar bursitis, or pain at the insertion of the quadriceps muscle or patellar tendon into the patella, may coexist with radiological evidence of mild OA which is not the cause of the pain. In this patient, medial joint compartment cartilage thinning and early osteophyte formation on the tibial and femoral medial joint margins were associated with pain on walking. This was not relieved by a local injection into a tender spot over the medial ligament, and early symptomatic OA was diagnosed. Although slightly limiting, the situation remained stable for several years before eventually requiring surgery. A spiked appearance to the tibial spines on X-ray is sometimes a sign of early OA, but it is of little clinical significance as an independent observation.

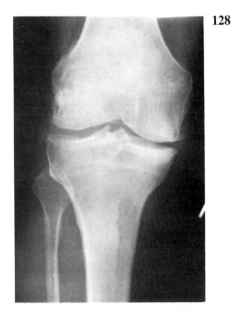

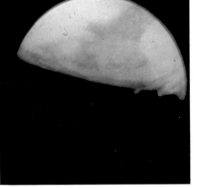

129 Arthroscopic appearances of early OA of the knee. The typical changes of OA can be clearly seen at arthroscopy. The cartilage is ulcerated and fragmented. At a later stage, the underlying bone becomes exposed and sclerotic.

130

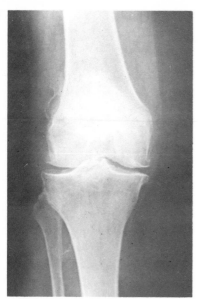

130 More advanced OA of the knee. Bilateral involvement, with narrowing of medial and lateral compartments and osteophyte formation on medial and lateral joint margins, is associated with more constant pain and marked stiffening after inactivity (gelling): the first steps after a period of rest are painful, but the discomfort decreases once the patient gets moving. This is a common complaint in symptomatic OA of weight-bearing joints. This patient should be encouraged to strengthen the quadriceps muscles and to use NSAIDs or analgesics judiciously, but only if they clearly help.

131

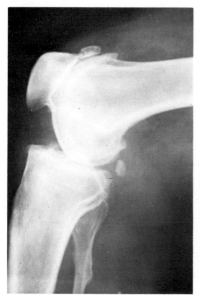

132

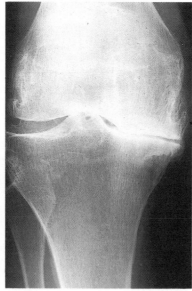

132 Severe OA of the knee. Once this degree of cartilage loss and osteophyte formation (here predominantly affecting the medial compartment) has occurred, NSAIDs and analgesics rarely alleviate pain experienced during weight-bearing. Pain at rest may also be severe. Joint replacement surgery should be considered as an appropriate measure to relieve discomfort and improve mobility (*see* Chapter 11).

131 Patellofemoral OA. This lateral view of the knee reveals marked reduction of the patellofemoral joint space, with osteophytes on the upper pole of the patella and the anterior surface of the femur. In some patients this develops in isolation, without involvement of the main tibiofemoral joint. Marked retropatellar creaking and pain on flexion and extension of the knee are very disabling. In cases of milder anterior knee pain, vigorous quadriceps muscle exercises are helpful because normal patellar function is highly dependent upon good quadriceps strength, and especially upon that of the vastus medialis muscle. Patellectomy may be indicated in an affected individual who has severe retropatellar pain but normal tibiofemoral joints. True locking of the knee (episodes of inability to straighten the flexed knee) may indicate an associated meniscal tear or loose intra-articular body, in which case arthroscopy should be considered. (The rounded opacity lying behind the knee in this X-ray is the fabella, a sesamoid bone (intratendinous centre of ossification), and is a normal finding.)

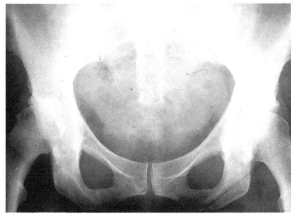

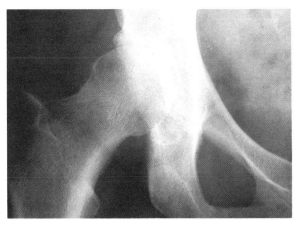

133 & 134 Early OA of the hip. The symptoms of early OA of the hip include pain in the groin, buttock and upper thigh, initially only when weight-bearing. Pain radiating to the knee is common and occasionally constitutes the main complaint. The hips should always be examined in patients with knee pain. The earliest physical finding is of pain, with restriction of internal rotation when the hip is held in flexion. The X-ray shows some narrowing of the articular cartilage at the upper pole of the femoral head, and sclerosis of the adjacent acetabulum which is dysplastic (shallow) (**134**). Occasionally, a more concentric patten of cartilage loss is seen; in such cases the reactive sclerosis distinguishes OA from an acute inflammatory arthritis, where such sclerosis is absent (*see* **53 & 187**). The patient may not be greatly troubled by pain at this stage, although stiffness may make reaching to the foot difficult, for example, when cutting toenails or putting on socks or stockings. Pain may be intermittent or episodic, possibly reflecting the occasional development of a transient joint effusion.

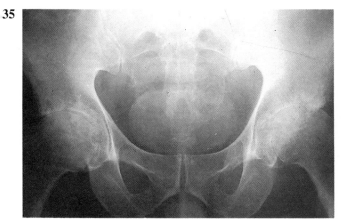

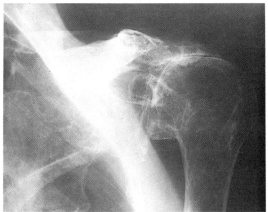

135 Advanced OA of the hip. In this patient a reactive cuff of osteophytes has formed around the femoral head. Pain sometimes waxes and wanes, so surgery should not be rushed into. However, when discomfort increases and resting pain that is no longer adequately controlled by drugs develops, or when stiffening becomes severely disabling, total hip replacement should be considered (*see* Chapter 11). This is a safe and successful solution for most patients. Cysts can here be seen in both femoral heads. Sudden worsening of symptoms may be due to the collapse of such a cyst.

136 OA of the shoulder. The shoulder is rarely affected by OA unless there has been predisposing trauma (a fracture of the head of the humerus or, as seen here, a chronic tear of the rotator cuff). The shoulder is occasionally affected in severe generalised OA. Pain, often severe at night, and restriction of movement may be very troublesome. A local corticosteroid injection can be administered, but it usually produces only temporary relief, or none at all. If this fails, a suprascapular nerve block, using a long-acting local anaesthetic such as bupivacaine, will occasionally give more prolonged relief. A total replacement of the shoulder alleviates pain, but rarely improves the range of movement. It remains a less satisfactory procedure than other joint replacements, and is best performed by an experienced surgeon with a specific interest in shoulder replacements.

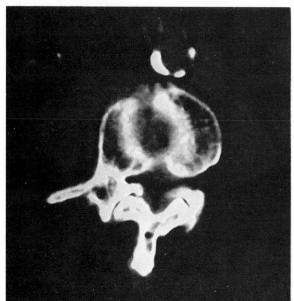

Front

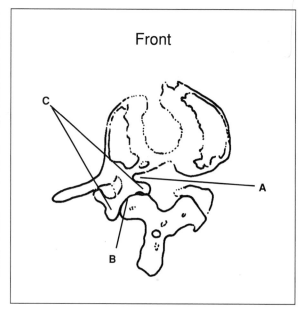

137 & 138 Spinal facet joint OA. In patients with severe spondylosis, narrowing of the disc space leads to misalignment of the posterior facet joints, which develop secondary OA. This may produce back pain which can be relieved by injecting the relevant joint under X-ray guidance. Occasionally, the resultant osteophytes impinge on the adjacent root canal, which has already been narrowed by the reduction in disc thickness, and the syndrome of spinal nerve root claudication may arise (*see*

170). With spinal nerve root claudication, the patient complains of pain and paraesthesia in the distribution of the affected root after walking (*see* **Table 11**, p.75), symptoms which are slowly relieved by rest. Computed tomography reveals the narrow root canal and striking osteophyte formation around the facet joints. A surgeon with an interest in back pain should be consulted. (A = root canal, B = facet joint, C = osteophytes.)

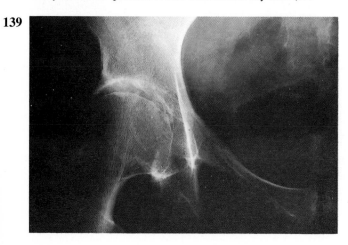

139 Secondary OA in a patient with acromegaly. Acromegaly may produce an increased thickness of cartilage and of soft tissues, and is thought to lead to OA in some patients. In this case the hip joint demonstrates a relatively normal joint space, but there are changes in the acetabulum and femoral head that resemble those of OA – sclerosis and marginal osteophyte formation. This patient, although asymptomatic, is at risk of developing symptomatic secondary OA at an early age. Control of the acromegaly does not appear to improve its associated joint problems (*see also* **286 & 287**). Other causes of secondary OA are listed in **Table 3**.

Management of osteoarthritis

There is a common misconception that osteoarthritis means inevitable pain and eventual disability. In English (but not in all languages) this reinforced by the use of the single word 'arthritis' to cover the whole spectrum of joint disease. All too often, this negative approach is adopted and reinforced by a medical profession which must learn to take a more positive view. Radiologically mild OA may be coincidental to the problem, and alternative causes of pain should be identified and treated. Even if the diagnosis is one of symptomatic OA, which is technically incurable, much can be done to alleviate unnecessary anxiety, reduce pain and improve function. In mild cases, nothing *need* be done, but this should be explained to patients positively, not simply as 'nothing *can* be done'. Locally applied heat, ice packs or various topical treatments are safe procedures which may be beneficial and should be encouraged. A general daily exercise programme and loss of excess weight are also important. Isometric, non weight-bearing exercises can be taught for specific joint problems: seek a physiotherapist's advice if patients need encouragement and motivation. Rest during acute flares, and the use of a walking stick or of a variety of resting splints, may be appropriate. The overall aim should be to help patients to cope better with their pain and to encourage them to remain as normally active as possible. Strenuous sports and heavy manual labour are best avoided, but, in general, patients should be reassured that tolerable pain during activity rarely means that they are doing themselves harm.

Although simple analgesics and/or NSAIDs can provide pain relief, it is rarely complete, weight-bearing pain, in particular, being difficult to alleviate. Side-effects act as an important curb on the indiscriminate use of these drugs, especially in the elderly, and have led to recent adverse publicity, which has heightened public awareness of the risks. The best approach is to discuss the most common side-effects and to encourage patients to use the drugs on a 'when necessary' basis, which may mean taking them before they go for a walk,

play golf or go shopping. If the drugs are needed regularly, patients should be encouraged to try to stop taking them from time to time to see if they are indeed still necessary and helpful. In elderly patients, especially those who are also taking diuretics, occasional checks of renal function should be performed. The evidence for specific NSAIDs either increasing joint damage or offering some form of local beneficial 'chondro-protective' effect remains conflicting.

Local corticosteroid injections into associated tender soft tissue lesions, or into joints that are inflamed or have an effusion, can be helpful, but they should not be repeated too often. Regional pain blocks may help temporarily.

Surgery (*see* Chapter 11) offers most patients the best hope of relief from intractable and disabling pain. In the younger patient it may be appropriate to consider whether osteotomy is feasible. Joint arthroplasty, whether replacement, interposition or excision, is now widely available and successful. Although the risks of infection or loosening of a joint replacement are slight, they are sufficient to justify trying other approaches first. In the younger patient, especially if they are otherwise fit and have single joint disease, the risk of subsequent loosening of a total hip or knee replacement is greater than that in the older patient or those whose activities are limited by polyarticular disease. Re-operation during the younger patient's remaining lifetime will probably be necessary. This knowledge often helps patients to keep going a little longer without surgery, but, if all else fails, replacement surgery has its place, even in the young. The use of noncemented hips in such circumstances remains controversial, but is increasingly beneficial (*see* Chapter 11).

With severe generalised osteoarthritis and with patients who are unfit for surgery or for whom surgery has failed, referral to a specialist pain clinic should be considered, and the advice of an occupational therapist and of social support services should be sought.

4 Crystal synovitis

Despite Garrod's suggestion in 1876 that the critical event in acute gout was the deposition of sodium urate crystals in the joints, it was only in the 1960s that examination of synovial fluid for crystals became routine in the investigation of acute arthritis. Two main crystal types, monosodium urate and calcium pyrophosphate, account for the majority of cases of crystal synovitis. They can be distinguished by their different appearance and their refringent properties under polarised light. In patients with gout, crystals are present in the joint fluid of noninflamed, asymptomatic joints. They cause an intense inflammatory response only when ingested by polymorphonuclear leucocytes, which then become activated and release the proinflammatory contents of their phagosomes into the joint. The trigger for this phagocytosis is still not fully understood, but it may require prior protein deposition on the crystals, intra-articular trauma or a sudden change in urate concentration (such as may occur when starting allopurinol treatment).

Gout

Uric acid is the end product of the metabolism of endogenous and dietary purines in humans, and cannot itself be metabolised further. It is normally excreted through the kidney (two-thirds) and the gut (one-third). Increased production of uric acid and/or failure of the kidneys to excrete it leads to hyperuricaemia. Blood levels of uric acid show a normal distribution in the population, with a skew towards the upper end of the range, reflecting those more susceptible to developing gout. Levels rise with age and are higher in men than women, especially before the female menopause. The majority of hyperuricaemic individuals are asymptomatic, being discovered only on routine biochemical screening. The ranges for gouty and normal individuals form two separate but overlapping distribution curves.

Acute gout is the most common presentation of hyperuricaemia. Other presentations include: tophaceous gout; renal colic due to uric acid stones; and chronic renal failure due to uric acid crystal deposition in the kidneys. Renal failure due to some other cause may lead to secondary hyperuricaemia.

Essential hyperuricaemia is sometimes familial, and presents symptomatically in young or middle-aged men. In some cases an abnormality of the kidney's complex mechanisms for handling uric acid, which leads to a reduced output of uric acid in the urine, can be demonstrated. In others the abnormality lies in the enzymes that metabolise purines, or in control of these enzymes, in which case there may be an abnormally high uric acid excretion in the urine, even on a purine-free diet. Secondary hyperuricaemia has a variety of different causes, the most common being renal impairment, due to essential hypertension, and the long-term use of thiazide or loop diuretics. These drugs are the most frequent cause of symptomatic hyperuricaemia in elderly women, who may develop acute mono- or polyarticular gout or tophaceous deposits. The rarer causes should be borne in mind when assessing any new case of symptomatic or asymptomatic hyperuricaemia, particularly if there is no family history, or if the patient is female or is otherwise atypical.

Lead poisoning, seen commonly until recently in plumbers or people working with lead paints, damages the renal tubules and leads to so-called 'saturnine gout', also known as 'pauper's gout'. The role of alcohol in precipitating gout is of historical importance: in the eighteenth and nineteenth centuries the main factor was probably that port was stored and transported in bottles made of lead glass, not in the usual wooden wine barrels, and consequently contained contained high levels of lead. Thus, so-called 'rich man's gout' may have been due to the same basic mechanism as pauper's gout! Other reasons include the high purine content of certain alcoholic drinks, especially beers, and a high calorie intake from regular drinking.

Table 6. Causes of secondary hyperuricaemia.

Increased uric acid production	Decrease of renal excretion
a) *Dietary* (offal, beer, etc. *see* **Table 8**)	a) *Impairment of renal tubular excretion of uric acid*
b) *Increased cell turnover*	Dehydration and/or starvation
Psoriasis (usually asymptomatic hyperuricaemia)	Essential hypertension
Lymphoproliferative disorders – Hodgkin's and	Drugs – thiazide and loop diuretics
other lymphomas	Low doses of aspirin
Myeloproliferative disorders – myeloma, leukaemias	Lead poisoning
Haemolytic anaemias	Diabetic ketoacidosis/lactic acidosis
Polycythaemia - primary or secondary	
Carcinomatosis	b) *Renal failure* – most commonly hypertensive
c) *Specific enzyme defects*	
HGPRT deficiency (Lesch–Nyhan disease)	

140   **141**   **142**

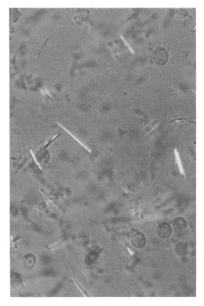
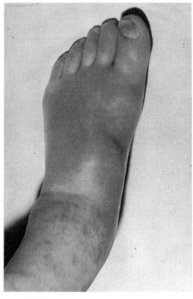
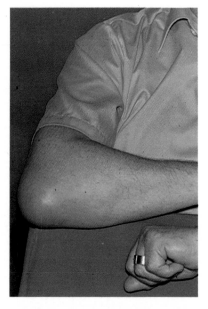

140 Monosodium urate crystals under polarised light. Crystals of either monosodium urate or calcium pyrophosphate may be found in synovial fluid samples during acute crystal synovitis. These needle-shaped crystals are typical of monosodium urate and demonstrate strong positive birefringence under polarised light with a red filter. This finding is diagnostic of acute gout.

141 Acute gout of the first MTP joint. About 70% of cases of acute gout present with very severe pain of the first MTP joint, which becomes hot, red, swollen and exquisitely tender. In this patient, there is also a marked inflammatory reaction of the whole foot (gouty cellulitis). The pain of acute gout is more severe than that of any other form of arthritis except for an acute infective arthritis or an acute haemoarthrosis, and these may need to be excluded by examination of the aspirate from the joint. An acute attack may be precipitated in susceptible subjects by surgery, dehydration, crash dieting or an alcoholic binge, or it may occur without apparent cause.

The finding of a raised blood uric acid level is usual. Aspiration of the first MTP joint is difficult, and rarely necessary in the typical case. It may be appropriate to aspirate the large joints for diagnostic purposes, and detection of monosodium urate crystals in synovial fluid is diagnostic. The fluid is always turbid, but not purulent, and contains large numbers of polymorphs on microscopy. Untreated, an attack will last 5–15 days. As the attack resolves, there is often slight peeling of the overlying skin.

Acute gouty polyarthritis is uncommon, but it is seen in patients on high doses of diuretics or in renal failure, and, occasionally, in patients started inappropriately on allopurinol treatment during or too soon after an acute attack (*see* p.63).

142 Acute gouty olecranon bursitis. This patient's gout presented for the first time as an acute olecranon bursitis, from which monosodium urate crystals were aspirated. Other bursae may also be affected.

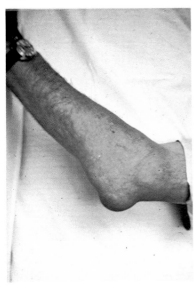
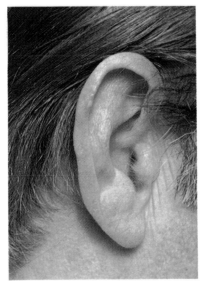
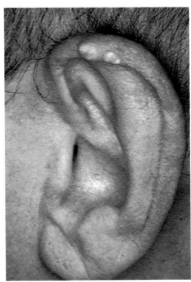

143 Chronic gouty olecranon bursitis. The presence of painless chronic bursitis, with crystals of uric acid obtained on aspiration, led to the recognition of incipient renal failure in this patient.

144 & 145 Typical gouty tophi. Painless, hard deposits of uric acid may be found over the pinna of the ear. The finding of such deposits in a patient presenting with an acute monoarthritis is strongly suggestive of gout. Removal of the deposits, which is not necessary, reveals typical urate crystals and/or more amorphous deposits.

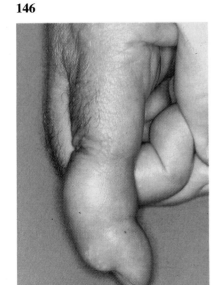
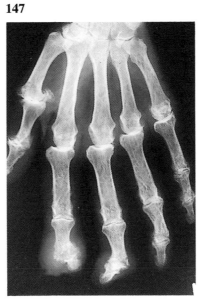
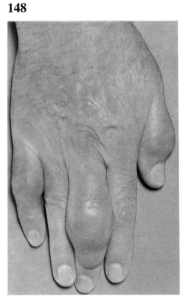

146 Chronic tophaceous gout. For reasons that remain unclear, not all gouty patients present with acute arthritis. Instead they present with tophi around the joints. These are either asymptomatic or lead to local stiffness, as in this patient with a large but painless deposit on the finger. The mottled white appearance is typical. Renal function should be investigated in such patients.

147 Radiological appearance of tophi. Tophaceous deposits can be distinguished from calcinosis (*see* **230 & 231**) by their radiological appearance. They are less radio-opaque than calcinotic deposits and are often described as giving a 'halo' effect, as demonstrated around the index and middle DIP joints of this patient.

148 Acute gout and chronic gouty arthritis. In this patient, acute polyarticular gout was superimposed on a background of chronic tophaceous swelling, and led to his presentation. He was on long-term diuretic treatment for heart failure.

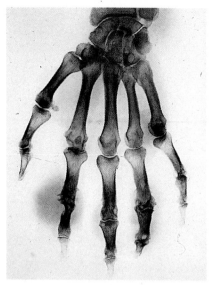 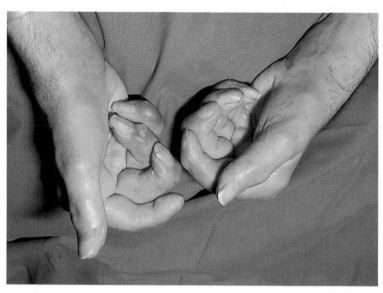

149 & 150 Severe chronic tophaceous gout. 149 shows tophaceous material, deposited most strikingly around the second PIP joint. Urate deposition in bone may produce a typical 'punched out' erosion of juxta-articular bone, here clearly visible in the middle phalanx of the index finger.

Occasionally, the presence of multiple deposits is associated with severe deformity, as in this patient (**150**) with chronic renal failure. His hands were also severely deformed, with multiple tophaceous deposits. The patient was a heavy drinker, showed poor compliance, and had developed marked renal impairment, all of which account for the unusual severity of the clinical picture. He also suffered acute gouty attacks which were difficult to control.

Management of acute gout

Acute attacks of gout should never be treated with allopurinol or a uricosuric agent. Although these drugs reduce the blood uric acid level, the resultant flux of urate from the tissues is likely to lead to further, perhaps even more painful or polyarticular attacks, causing patients to lose faith in the drug. Allopurinol-induced acute gout is one of the rare situations in which gout can be diagnosed despite a normal serum uric acid level.

The patient with acute gout is in severe pain. In some cases it is warranted to start treatment with an intramuscular injection of an **NSAID**. Most patients respond well to an oral preparation such as indomethacin, naproxen or diclofenac, given in initially high doses with food, and then in normal doses at regular intervals once the pain has subsided (*see* **Table 7**). Treatment ideally should be maintained for at least one week after the attack has settled fully. In patients who have a history of peptic ulceration or renal failure, it is safer to use **colchicine**: an initial dose of 1 mg is followed by a further 1 mg after 4–6 hours, and then by 1 mg every 6–8 hours until pain control is achieved, at which point the dose can be reduced to 0.5 mg every 8 hours. Although these doses may produce abdominal colic or diarrhoea, they are less likely to than is the traditional approach of giving 0.5 mg every 2 hours, which should not be employed.

Occasionally, acute attacks are difficult to control and require a combination of an NSAID and colchicine.

A single attack of gout, particularly one precipitated by unusual stress such as recent surgery, does not require long-term drug management. Dietary advice (*see* **Table 8**), a considerable reduction in alcohol consumption, weight loss and control of hypertension are worthwhile, and it may be necessary to consider stopping thiazide diuretics and using other hypotensive agents if they are needed. These approaches may delay further attacks or, occasionally, halt the problem completely.

Table 7. NSAID doses for the treatment of acute gout.

Indomethacin	75 mg immediately, then 50 mg every 6–8 hours, then 25 mg every 8 hours
Naproxen	750 mg immediately, then 500 mg every 6–8 hours, then 250 mg every 8 hours
Diclofenac	75 mg immediately, then 50 mg every 6–8 hours, then 25 mg every 8 hours
All should be administered with food	

Table 8. Some foods to avoid in hyperuricaemia.

Offal	Heart, kidney, liver, sweetbreads (pancreas)
Fish	Anchovies, herrings, mackerel, salmon, shellfish
Vegetables	Spinach
Other meats and fish may be eaten in moderation	

Management of recurrent gout and of tophaceous gout

Some patients require longer-term drug management. The use of allopurinol (a xanthine oxidase inhibitor which reduces uric acid production) or, less commonly, of a uricosuric agent such as probenecid, is necessary to control frequent attacks of acute gout, or if polyarticular gout occurs. The presence of tophi or of gross hyperuricaemia of more than 700 μmol/l in the younger, asymptomatic patient with a family history of gout also indicates the use of these drugs. In addition, the dietary and other general measures described above should be introduced. In renal failure, allopurinol should be used, but at a lower dose as it is renally excreted. In such cases, and if there is a history of uric acid renal stone formation, uricosuric agents are contraindicated.

Allopurinol should never be started, nor the dose increased, during or within six weeks of an acute attack of gout, as it may cause a severe flare It should always be introduced under the cover of regular daily doses of either an NSAID or colchicine for the first six weeks, to prevent it from precipitating an attack. The standard dose is 300 mg daily, but some patients may need up to 600 mg. In those with renal impairment, 50–100 mg should be prescribed, and renal function checked regularly. In addition to lowering serum uric acid levels, this drug also produces a gradual reduction of tophaceous deposits. Despite the need to use it over long periods, allopurinol is a safe drug (a few patients develop an allergic rash). The risk of side-effects due to allopurinol is greater in patients with renal disease or diuretic-induced hyperuricaemia. If gout recurs despite adequate treatment, it is likely that the patient is still drinking alcohol to excess.

Uricosuric agents, the most widely available of which are probenecid (0.5–2 g daily) and sulphinpyrazone (50–400 mg daily), act by increasing the renal excretion of uric acid. Alkalinisation of the urine may prevent the precipitation of urate in the kidney, but these agents should be avoided if renal disease is present or suspected. Since the introduction of allopurinol, they are mainly used as a supplement in the rare patient whose attacks cannot be controlled by allopurinol alone; in severe tophaceous gout, again in combination with allopurinol; or alone in patients allergic to allopurinol.

Chondrocalcinosis and acute pseudogout

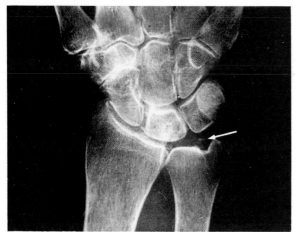

151

Table 9. Clinical patterns of chrondrocalcinosis.

Asymptomatic
Acute pseudogout
Pseudo-osteoarthritis (±acute pseudogout)
Pseudorheumatoid arthritis

151 Chondrocalcinosis of the wrist. After the knee, the wrist is the most commonly affected joint, with deposits usually appearing in the triangular ligament (arrow). In younger patients who demonstrate symptomatic or asymptomatic chondrocalcinosis on X-rays, associated diseases such as hyperparathyroidism, haemochromatosis or hypothyroidism should be excluded.

152

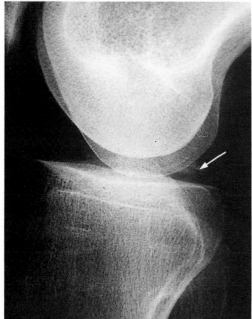

153

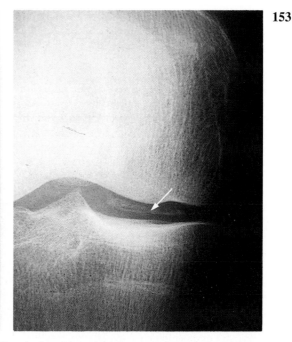

152 & 153 Typical chondrocalcinosis of the knee. Chronic deposition of calcium pyrophosphate in cartilage is observed on X-rays more frequently with increasing age, reaching an incidence of more than 5% in those over 70 years. It is usually asymptomatic, but may coexist with radiological changes of OA (*see* **156 & 157**). Deposition occurs both in the fibrocartilaginous menisci (as here) and in the hyaline cartilage. The latter produces a fine line of calcification parallel to the surface of the bone, which can be best seen in the lateral view, running around the femoral condyle (*see* **157**).

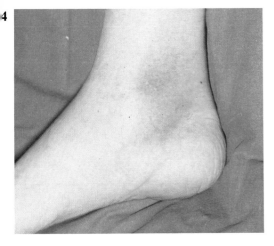

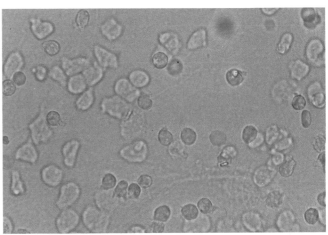

154 Acute pseudogout of the ankle. One in four patients with symptomatic chondrocalcinosis develops episodic attacks of acute inflammatory arthritis with severe pain, redness and swelling. The clinical picture mimics acute urate gout, although it usually affects the wrist, knee or ankle. It may be polyarticular. Attacks are spontaneous, or precipitated by surgery or an acute illness; untreated, they last about two weeks. They are often associated with fever and a leucocytosis, and infective arthritis is an important differential diagnosis. If in doubt, refer to a specialist for aspiration of the joint. The fluid should always be sent for culture and Gram staining, as well as being examined by polarised light microscopy.

155 Crystals of calcium pyrophosphate from a joint affected by acute pseudogout. Examination of the joint fluid reveals rhomboidal, weakly positively birefringent intra- and extracellular crystals of calcium pyrophosphate. They are smaller and more difficult to see than the crystals of monosodium urate. The cause of shedding of the calcium pyrophosphate crystals into the joint is not known. They do not always cause acute inflammation. (Occasionally, gout occurs coincidentally with chrondrocalcinosis and can be recognised by the presence of needle-shaped, strongly negatively birefringent crystals of monosodium urate.)

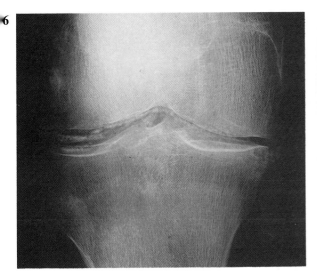

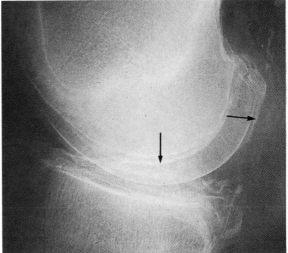

156 & 157 OA complicating chondrocalcinosis. This man had marked chondrocalcinosis which led to the early development of OA in the affected knee. Chondrocalcinosis in the hyaline cartilage can be seen in the lateral view (arrows). In a few cases, chondrocalcinosis is associated with a particularly destructive variant of OA, which affects a different pattern of joints from that in typical generalised OA (*see* p.49). This is sometimes called pseudo-osteoarthritis: the knees, wrists, MCP joints, hips and shoulders are affected in decreasing order of frequency. (About 5% of patients with widespread chondrocalcinosis have a chronic inflammatory arthritis which mimics RA.)

Management of acute pseudogout

Attacks respond well to therapeutic aspiration of the joint, combined with the use of NSAIDs, initially in high doses. Colchicine, which is safer in patients with a history of peptic ulceration, is also effective. If infection can be safely discounted, an intra-articular or intramuscular corticosteroid injection can be used for a very painful attack. In recurrent attacks, repeated aspiration is not necessary unless drug therapy is unsuccessful. Continuous doses of an NSAID or of colchicine may be needed occasionally as a preventive measure in severe cases. Allopurinol is ineffective. Pseudo-osteoarthritis and pseudorheumatoid arthritis are best managed symptomatically.

5 Spinal disorders

The spine is a structure of great complexity, comprising bone, fibrous joints (discs), synovial joints (facets), ligaments, muscles and nerves. This complexity explains why many of the problems that arise in and around the spine, especially the majority of mechanical spinal disorders, are poorly understood. Usually precipitated by injudicious movements or trauma, many are self-limiting and improve with analgesia, brief periods of rest and the passage of time. They are rarely, if ever, seen by a doctor and settle spontaneously, or with the help of a physiotherapist or an osteopath. Such problems are, however, a major cause of time off work in most industrialised countries and, despite attempts to improve working conditions, commonly arise as workplace injuries.

The main symptom of uncomplicated mechanical spinal syndromes is painful restriction of spinal movements, occasionally associated with the development of an inability to make certain specific movements, or of a fixed abnormal position (such as that seen in acute torticollis). Generally, the pain is localised, but it may radiate distally. It tends to be associated with painful secondary muscle spasm, which worsens if treatment is delayed. This spasm may affect a wider area than that of the initial problem, thus producing more diffuse discomfort. There may be maximal tenderness at the site of the primary lesion, but the tenderness is often also diffuse. Some of these mechanical episodes respond to manipulative therapy. Although usually short-lived, they can recur or develop into a more chronic back or neck syndrome, requiring further investigation and expert management. Chronic spinal pain can lead to anxiety, irritability and depression, sometimes becoming the main manifestation of an underlying psychosocial problem.

Certain features of pain arising from the spine indicate that a more serious problem may be present:

- Pain radiating down an arm or leg, with associated paraesthesia, numbness or weakness, suggests nerve root irritation, due either to an acute disc prolapse or to root canal narrowing that is caused by spondylotic changes and/or secondary facet joint OA (*see* **137 & 138**). X-rays are obligatory with such symptoms, particularly to exclude structural damage after major trauma.
- Night pain, associated with morning stiffness that is eased by exercise, indicates an inflammatory problem such as ankylosing spondylitis (see p.78). However, mechanical spinal pain can also be worse in the morning if a poor bed or inappropriate pillows are used.
- Unremitting pain, which is worse at night and associated with systemic illness, suggests a primary or secondary tumour or an infective lesion. Pain in the midline in the thoracic spine is frequently serious and warrants investigation to rule out malignancy or infection.
- In elderly patients with osteoporosis, wedge fractures of the dorsal or lumbar vertebrae may occur spontaneously or after minimal trauma. They produce severe local pain which is initially little eased by rest, but settles over 4–6 weeks. A wedge fracture should always be viewed as suspicious of an underlying primary or secondary malignancy, and warrants further investigation. X-rays, a bone scan or an MRI scan may be necessary to exclude such a problem, and a needle biopsy may be indicated.
- Rarely, back pain is referred from an intra-abdominal cause, such as a penetrating posterior duodenal ulcer, renal or pancreatic lesions, or a lesion of the pleura, in which cases other symptoms may be present.

If these more serious problems are not to be missed, a careful history and examination are essential in all cases, especially when these atypical features are elicited.

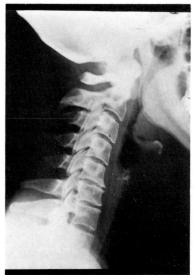

158 Insignificant cervical spondylotic changes. Narrowing of the C5/6 and C6/7 discs is here associated with minor osteophytic changes of the anterior border on the adjacent vertebrae at C5/6. Such appearances are common after 40 years of age, only rarely causing symptoms. The radiological changes cannot be altered by treatment, although episodes of pain, which arise coincidentally from muscles or from some other soft-tissue cause, generally settle. Such patients should not be told that they have 'arthritis of the spine' or 'degeneration of the spine', as such news causes unnecessary anxiety and implies a worse outlook than is usually the case. The loss of normal cervical lordosis in this X-ray merely indicates that the patient is in pain and has spasm of the neck muscles.

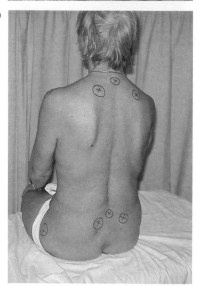

159 Neck pain and tender paracervical trigger points. The most common cause of neck pain is muscular; it is often precipitated by poor posture (working at a desk that is too low, or sitting with work in the lap and with the neck flexed awkwardly for long periods) or by muscle spasm. Muscle spasm may initially be secondary to the pain of an acute mechanical problem, but it is often perpetuated by stress and anxiety. A cycle of pain and spasm can be set up, rendering the problem chronic, and increasing a patient's sense of stress. Such patients frequently have tender trigger points over one or both trapezius muscles, over the spinous process of C7, over the paracervical muscles and/or along the occipital ridge. Muscle spasm is often visible: the shoulder(s) may be elevated or the neck muscles prominent. Some patients also experience typical muscle tension headaches and complain of occipital and bitemporal pain, usually described as feeling like 'pressure' or a 'tight band around the head'. Analgesia, physiotherapy and explanation and reassurance help recovery. Attention to sleeping position and the provision of a firm bed are also beneficial. Relaxation techniques, together with modifications of working positions and practices, may help to prevent recurrences. In addition to the trigger points in the cervical region, this patient had similar tender spots in the lumbar region and suffered chronic low back pain (*see also* **169** & **Fibromyalgia**, p.155).

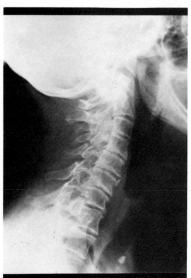

160 Midcervical spondylosis. The more advanced changes seen on this X-ray may be asymptomatic or associated with symmetrical stiffening of the neck; difficulty in looking behind when reversing the car is a common complaint. Cracking or creaking, audible to the patient on movement, is worrying but not usually important. Acute episodes of neck pain may occur and are relieved by analgesia, the use of a collar for short periods, and physiotherapy.

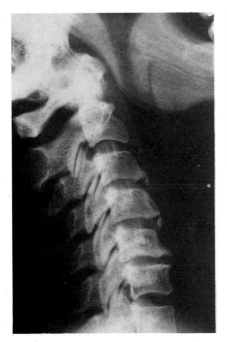
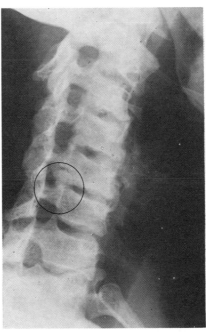

161 & 162 C6 nerve root compression by spondylotic osteophytes at C5/6. In more severe spondylosis, there may also be posterior osteophytes which may project into and narrow the canal and thus impinge on the emerging nerve root. This causes severe arm pain, with paraesthesia and numbness in the distribution of the affected nerve root. Neck pain is sometimes absent, but neck movements exacerbate the arm pain, suggesting the diagnosis. Plain lateral cervical spine films reveal anterior and posterior osteophytes at C5/6, but oblique X-ray views of the cervical spine are needed to confirm osteophytic encroachment into the root canal, at the level which correlates with the symptoms. This patient experienced paraesthesia in the thumb and index finger and had an absent biceps reflex, reduced supinator reflex and loss of biceps power. (The acute attack may be precipitated by a disc prolapse at the same level.) It is clearly important that the clinical findings are consistent with the level of radiological involvement. If this is not the case, further investigation is required.

The pain may be severe and is best treated with analgesia, rest in a soft cervical collar, support of the arm, and avoidance of lifting. Gentle intermittent traction from an experienced physiotherapist may be helpful. Surgical root canal decompression is only occasionally necessary.

Table 10. Symptoms and signs of cervical root compression.

Root	Disc level	Reflex reduced	Loss of power
C5	C4/5	(Biceps)	Shoulder
C6	C5/6	Biceps / Brachioradialis	Biceps Wrist extension
C7	C6/7	Triceps	Triceps
C8	C7/T1	(Triceps)	Intrinsic muscles of the hand

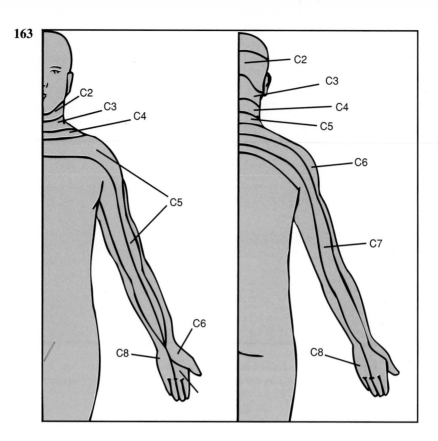

163 The dermatomal distribution of pain and paraesthesia in the arm.

Acute cervical disc prolapse

An acute cervical disc prolapse presents with a history of a sudden onset of diffuse neck pain, which radiates out to one shoulder and to the medial border of the scapula. Neck movements are asymmetrically reduced. Although the pain may settle, it usually progresses, after a variable delay, to severe, lancinating arm pain, and paraesthesia and numbness in a single nerve root distribution. Management should include a soft collar, supporting the affected arm in a sling, and adequate analgesia and muscle relaxants. The patient should rest and avoid carrying loads until the pain and sensory symptoms have resolved. If improvement is slow, surgical referral is indicated.

Shoulder pain radiating to the arm

Shoulder pain radiating to the arm is frequently misdiagnosed as pain arising from the neck. Generally, it can easily be distinguished by the fact that the arm pain is increased when the shoulder is moved, but not with movements of the neck. There may be also obvious restriction of shoulder movement (*see* **328–330**). Conversely, if the pain in the arm is due to nerve root irritation, shoulder movements are rarely painful or restricted, but the neck is restricted and movements may cause pain and/or paraesthesia in the arm.

164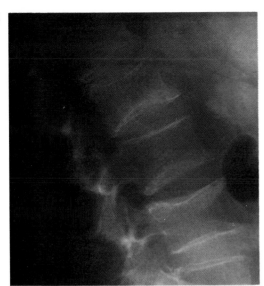

164–166 Osteoporotic crush fracture. This patient, on corticosteroids for polymyalgia rheumatica, suffered severe, episodic thoracolumbar pain, which radiated around the lower ribs during some attacks. The very severe pain lasted several weeks, necessitating bedrest and analgesia. Care must be taken to prevent the severe constipation that often develops during bedrest in the elderly, due to the combination of immobility and analgesia. The patient eventually developed a severe dorsal kyphosis due to multiple wedge fractures. In the lateral X-ray (**164**), T12 shows marked wedging, and endplate fractures affecting the upper lumbar vertebrae are also visible. The pedicles of the collapsed vertebra are intact on the anteroposterior view (**165**), a helpful factor in distinguishing this appearance from that of acute spinal collapse due to multiple metastatic deposits (*see* **167 & 168**).

165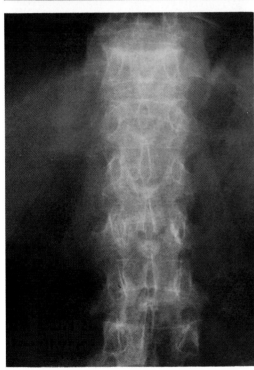

166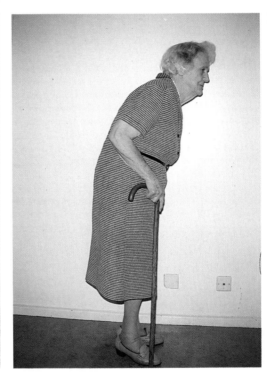

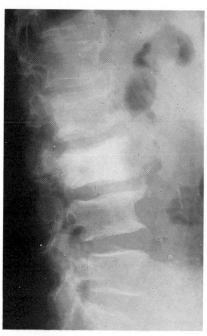
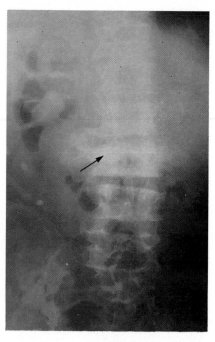

167 & 168 Spinal collapse due to malignancy. There may be a preceding history of localised back pain which worsens at night, or evidence of systemic disease: weight loss, malaise, fever, or a past history of treatment for a primary tumour elsewhere. Acute vertebral collapse is, however, a not uncommon first presentation of bony secondary deposits or of myeloma, in which case the pain is usually severe and of sudden onset. The diagnosis can generally be suspected from the clinical picture. X-rays demonstrate a localised collapse, without evidence of generalised osteoporosis. Here the vertebra is in fact sclerotic. An important clue may be seen on the anteroposterior film of the spine (**168**), where a pedicle has been destroyed (arrow). This loss of outline of the pedicle does not occur in osteoporotic spinal collapse. The primary malignancy may be found on general examination, but if detection proves difficult, it is a reasonably straightforward procedure to obtain a needle biopsy of the affected vertebra, using radiological screening to direct the needle. In most cases of collapse due to malignancy the extreme pain is rapidly relieved by local radiotherapy. The further management and outlook depend upon the specific cause, but the prognosis is generally poor. (*N.B.* This patient also has florid anterior bridging osteophytes with relatively normal discs – these are the appearances of ankylosing hyperostosis).

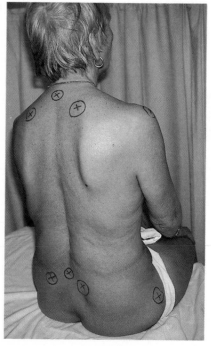

169 Fibrositic nodulosis. Fibrofatty nodules are frequently palpable across the iliac crests and over the sacroiliac joints. They are of no significance unless they are tender. They may cause pain which radiates from the buttock, down the back of the thigh and, occasionally, as far as the knee. Superficially, the pain mimics sciatica, but it is rarely as acute and is never associated with paraesthesia. A local injection of 25 mg hydrocortisone acetate into the nodule frequently resolves the problem. Such patients often have evidence of mild radiological spondylosis, but this is of no significance. As with this patient, there may be other tender trigger points (*see* **159** and p.155).

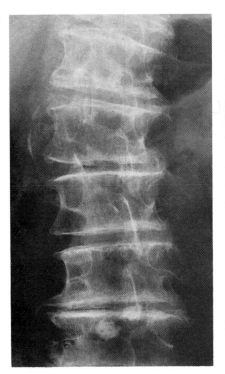 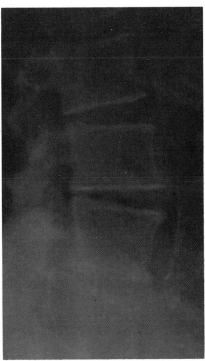

170 Severe lumbar spondylosis with a secondary scoliosis. Even in the presence of severe spondylotic changes and a secondary scoliosis, patients are not necessarily troubled by pain. Although spinal stiffening may develop, its insidious onset helps the individual to cope without much difficulty, When pain does occur, it may be acute and presumably traumatic, or chronic. It may be necessary to try a variety of different therapeutic approaches including intermittent or regular analgesia or NSAIDs, a lumbar support corset, and episodes of physiotherapy or osteopathy. Local corticosteroid injections into painful ligaments or into facet joints, the latter under radiological screening, may also offer relief. If the condition is chronically symptomatic, coming to terms with the problem is essential, however difficult. If all else fails, the patient may be helped by referral to a specialist pain clinic for behavioural psychology and other approaches.

This patient was pain-free until she developed acute right L5 root claudication, causing pain and paraesthesia in an L5 distribution, which were precipitated by walking and eased gradually by rest (compare **137 & 138**). (The paraesthesia and the slower relief of pain with rest distinguish this type of claudication from the more common form, which is due to impaired arterial circulation.) Her peripheral pulses were normal. Several weeks of bed rest relieved the pain and improved her walking distance.

171 Spondylolisthesis at L4/5. This X-ray demonstrates a forward slip of L4 on L5. In this case it was secondary to degenerative changes in the facet joints at this level. The appearances may be asymptomatic or associated with back pain or, occasionally, with nerve root pain (sometimes worse at night or when walking). If conservative approaches such as bedrest, a corset or physiotherapy fail, an expert surgical opinion should be sought, to consider spinal fusion at the affected level. In younger patients a spondylolisthesis is generally associated with bilateral congenital failure of fusion of the pars interarticularis at the affected level, in which case a pars defect can be best seen on an oblique view of the lumbar spine. Symptoms arising from a spondylolisthesis in a patient under 30 should be routinely be referred to a surgeon as fusion may be needed.

Spinal stenosis: a patient who complains of symmetrical pain and sensory symptoms that are brought on by walking may have spinal canal stenosis. In this syndrome the cauda equina is compromised by narrowing of the spinal canal. Patients often find that their pain is less severe when they walk with the lumbar spine flexed. This is because the anteroposterior width of the spinal canal is increased by flexion. For the same reason, bicycling does not produce the pain. The syndrome is commonly caused by a combination of a congenitally small anteroposterior lumbar canal width, with acquired narrowing due to severe posterior osteophyte formation, and/or a spondylolisthesis. Surgical canal decompression laminectomy is usually the management of choice.

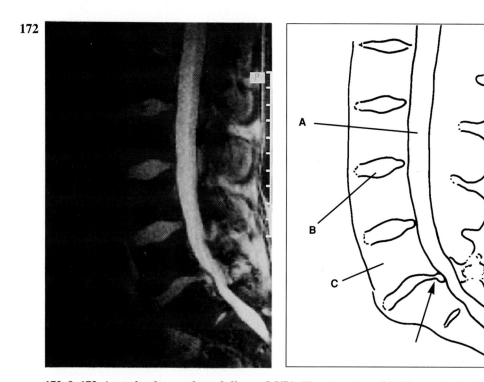

172 & 173 Acute lumbar prolapsed disc at L5/S1. The advantage of MRI scanning is that it is noninvasive. However, it is not yet widely available and remains costly. This sagittal view demonstrates a prolapse of the lumbosacral disc. A transverse view revealed that the disc was prolapsed to the right and pressing on the right S1 nerve root (arrow). The patient presented with severe right-sided back pain and radiation of acute pain to the lateral border of the right foot, where there was numbness. On examination, weakness of plantar flexion and loss of the right ankle reflex were also detected. Conservative treatment, with bed rest and adequate analgesia at home, was not effective. A 10-day inpatient stay and an epidural corticosteroid injection were also ineffective, and a surgical microdiscectomy was eventually required. It is essential to use a gradual therapeutic approach, only employing surgery when it is clear that other methods have failed: surgery relieves the leg pain in most cases, but some individuals may develop persistent back pain. Although this may well have occurred without surgical intervention, surgery may be blamed, and a general feeling of discontent and longer-term problems can arise. Most patients who are later dissatisfied with the outcome of their spinal surgery prove to have received insufficient prior conservative treatment or inadequate advice on what benefits and problems to expect after the procedure. (A = spinal canal, B = vertebral disc, C =vertebral body.)

Table 11. Symptoms and signs of lumbar root compression.

Root	Disc level	Reflex reduced	Loss of power
L3	L2/3	None	Hip flexion
L4	L3/4	Knee reflex	Quadriceps
L5	L4/5	None	Dorsiflexion of ankle/great toe
S1	L5/S1	Ankle reflex	Plantar flexion of ankle

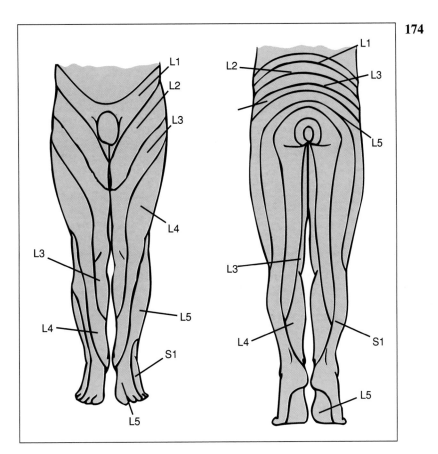

174 The dermatomal distribution of pain and paraesthesia in the leg.

Caution – central lumbar disc prolapse

If a prolapsed disc is suspected, it is essential to check that there is no loss of sensation in the perianal region, no loss of sensation or control when passing faeces, no loss of anal sphincter tone and no difficulty when passing urine. Any of these might imply a central disc prolapse, with compression of the cauda equina. This is a neurosurgical emergency, requiring urgent referral to prevent possible permanent loss of urethral and/or rectal control.

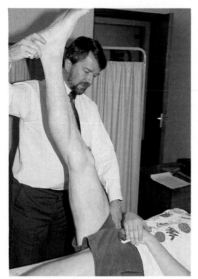

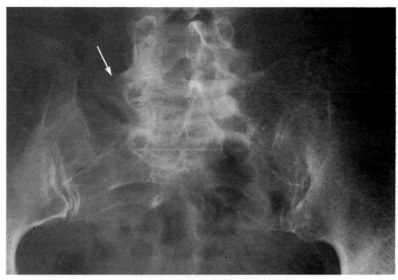

175 Straight-leg-raising test and femoral stretch test. Not all pain radiating from the lumbar spine to the leg is due to nerve root compression; it may simply reflect radiating pain. Paraesthesia and/or numbness associated with the pain are important historical findings which suggest neurological impingement. This can be confirmed by performing the straight-leg-raising test and femoral stretch tests. For the former test (**175**), patients should be supine. If they develop acute pain in the leg when the leg is raised with the knee straight to between 30 and 50° above horizontal (or less), the test is positive, indicating a probable impingement of the S1 or L5 root. Dorsiflexion of the foot, with the leg raised to the highest point, may increase the leg pain – a positive sciatic stretch test, again indicating probable nerve root impingement. With true acute S1 or L5 nerve root impingement, the straightened leg can rarely be raised beyond 50°. Pain produced at the back of the thigh or in the

back during the straight-leg-raising test is generally nonspecific.

For a higher lumbar root, the femoral stretch test is positive if severe pain is produced in the front of the thigh *of the affected side* when the patient lies prone and the leg is flexed at the knee.

176 Hemisacralisation of L5. L5 is asymmetrical on this X-ray, with a normal lumbar transverse process on one side (arrow), but fusion with the sacrum on the other . This relatively common spinal anomaly is usually of no clinical significance. Occasionally, however, such individuals are troubled by recurrent episodes of low back pain. A local corticosteroid injection may help, but patients generally have to learn back-strengthening exercises and specific techniques for lifting that avoid placing strain on the back. They may also have to avoid some sports, such as squash and tennis, which involve twisting and bending.

Management

The key to effective treatment of low back pain is diagnosis, although this remains an imprecise art. The simpler mechanical problems may be acutely painful, but they are rarely long-lived. Adequate analgesia, sensible advice about what to do and what to avoid, and a *brief* period of rest on a firm bed for low back pain, or in a collar for cervical pain, are usually sufficient. A physiotherapist or osteopath may help some of the more acute problems, but the clinician must feel confident that no more sinister, underlying cause exists, before the patient

is referred. A positive attitude, explanation and reassurance are all important and can prevent the problem becoming chronic. Friction in the workplace, with a lack of sympathy from employers, or a refusal to improve working conditions in response to the problem, may lead to longer-term difficulties and litigation. It is sometimes helpful for the doctor to speak directly to the employer.

The treatment of the more specific causes of back pain is dealt with under their respective headings.

6 Seronegative spondarthritides

The cumbersome title 'seronegative spondarthritis' is used to describe an assortment of conditions affecting the spine and peripheral joints, which have been observed to aggregate in family groups. Although the histology of the associated joint synovitis is difficult to distinguish from that of RA if routine techniques are used, differences are emerging which suggest that these diseases are triggered by micro-organisms or fragments of micro-organisms. Of historic importance in the recognition of these conditions was the observation that the patients are routinely seronegative for rheumatoid factor (hence the collective title). The diseases include ankylosing spondylitis (AS), psoriatic arthritis, reactive arthritis (Reiter's syndrome) and enteropathic arthritis (associated with ulcerative colitis and Crohn's disease). All are linked by an increased frequency of HLA B27 and a higher incidence of sacroiliitis than that seen in the general population. Several overlapping nonarticular problems are also seen; thus, uveitis is seen in all, the cutaneous lesions of reactive arthritis are histologically identical to those of pustular psoriasis, nail dystrophy occurs in psoriasis and reactive arthritis, and aortitis is occasionally seen in AS and reactive arthritis.

The common aetiopathogenetic thread of these disorders is yet to be unravelled. When the striking association of HLA B27 with AS was first demonstrated (present in more than 90% of Caucasians with the disease, but in only 8% of the control population) hopes were high. However, there is no demonstrably significant difference between the molecular structure of the gene in patients with AS and that of the gene in nonaffected HLA B27-positive individuals, although control of the expression of the gene on the cell surface may differ. A different line of research is beginning to suggest that molecular mimicry may be important in triggering these disorders, the idea being that the surface of an organism or some of its subunits may induce an antibody response. The resultant antibodies may then crossreact with the HLA B27 molecule. In AS, there are certainly detectable levels of antibodies which react with both HLA B27 and *Klebsiella* spp. (a commensal organism commonly found in the gut). Such antibodies are found less frequently in controls. If and how this reaction triggers disease is yet to be demonstrated. In Reiter's disease an association with a triggering infection is well established clinically, and intracellular fragments of *Chlamydia trachomatis*, one of the triggering organisms, have recently been demonstrated in the affected joints of some patients (*see* **209**). These fragments do not contain DNA, but are composed of lipopolysaccharides. The mucous membranes of the gut and the genitourinary tract, together with abnormalities of their defences, may also be important in causing or controlling these diseases and their manifestations. Much exciting work is still to be done, but current studies may open the door to understanding, eventually leading to more effective therapies and preventive measures.

These diseases may present in childhood, when the picture is often subtly different (*see* Chapter 8).

A brief family history inquiring specifically about spinal problems or the other manifestations of seronegative spondarthritis is mandatory in all individuals with recurrent back pain which is worse after rest, and in those with an unexplained inflammatory arthritis.

Ankylosing spondylitis

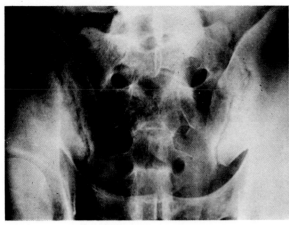

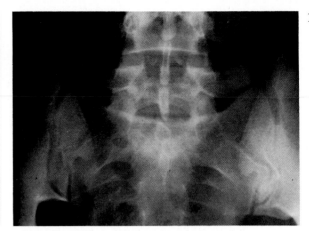

17

177 & 178 Early radiological sacroiliitis. Sacroiliac joint involvement is usually the first manifestation of ankylosing spondylitis, starting in the patient's late teens or early twenties. The initial complaint is of bouts of pain in one or both buttocks, sometimes accompanied by low back pain and stiffness. The pain and stiffness are typically worse in the morning and at night, being relieved by exercise. The bouts last from a few days to several months. Between bouts, at least initially, the patient is asymptomatic. During the first few years, radiological abnormalities are not seen. The diagnosis is often made after a delay of several years, either after one of the non-spinal complications such as uveitis or costochondritis supervenes, or when the persistence of the attacks leads to an X-ray or a specialist consultation. In this patient (**177**) the sacroiliac joints show early radiological changes. There is loss of definition of the cortical margins in their lower portions, and sclerosis affecting both the sacral and the iliac sides of the joints. An X-ray of normal sacroiliac joints is shown for comparison (**178**).

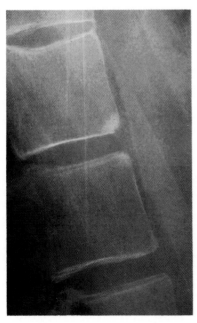

179 Early spinal lesion in AS. Spinal pain and stiffness often start insidiously. Unless the problem is correctly diagnosed and a combination of NSAIDs and a regular spinal mobilising exercise regime introduced, there is a risk that the spine will stiffen permanently. The earliest radiological appearance in the spine is a squaring of the normally concave anterior border of the lumbar vertebrae. This is due to blunting and blurring of the adjacent upper or lower discovertebral rim. If there is extensive bone erosion at this site, it is called a Romanus lesion. The inflammatory process responsible starts at the insertion of the intervertebral ligament into the vertebral margin, causing local

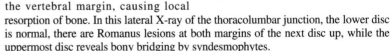

resorption of bone. In this lateral X-ray of the thoracolumbar junction, the lower disc is normal, there are Romanus lesions at both margins of the next disc up, while the uppermost disc reveals bony bridging by syndesmophytes.

180 More advanced disease with syndesmophyte formation. In AS the inflammatory lesions at the insertion of the intervertebral ligament heal by ossification. Untreated, this latter process may, in turn, lead to the development of intervertebral bony bridges or syndesmophytes, which follow the line of the intervertebral ligaments and usually bridge normal disc spaces. (Compare the narrowed disc space and 'beak' osteophytes of spondylosis (*see* **170**)). Radiologically, the thoracolumbar region of the spine is often affected first. As this is easily missed on standard lumbar spine views, extended views which include the thoracolumbar junction, or specific views of that area should be requested.

181 Andersson lesion. This type of discovertebral lesion is sometimes seen in AS, and may lead to anxiety about the possibility of an infective discitis. The lesions may form centrally in the vertebra or, as here, peripherally, and probably reflect local osteoporosis due to the inflammatory process with secondary disc herniation.

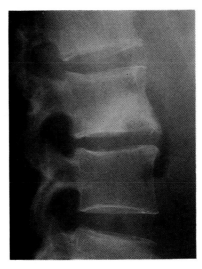

181

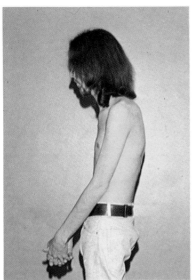

182

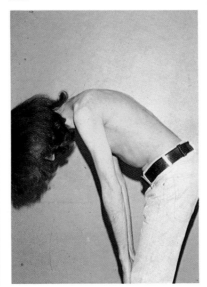

183

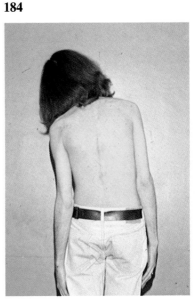

184

182–184 Spinal stiffening and paraspinal muscle wasting in AS. During painful episodes early in the disease, the patient becomes stooped and there is reversible stiffening of the spine, which can be relieved by NSAIDs and exercise. If syndesmophyte formation is extensive, however, the stiffening becomes irreversible, and marked paraspinal muscle wasting may develop. The dorsal kyphosis becomes fixed, forward flexion is limited to movements at the hips, and lateral flexion is severely restricted. Marked paraspinal muscle wasting is apparent. At this stage, it is essential that neck movements are maintained and that any increase in the dorsal kyphosis is prevented by regular exercises.

Involvement of the thoracic spine and of the costovertebral joints leads to restriction of chest expansion, which should be measured regularly. Restriction can be prevented by regular deep-breathing exercises. However, if costovertebral joint fusion occurs, the patient develops abdominal protrusion and breathes using the abdominal muscles. Costochondral joint inflammation may produce anterior chest discomfort, and is a further cause of painful restriction of chest expansion. Inflammation may affect one or many costochondral junctions. Rarely, and probably because of restricted expansion, upper lobe lung fibrosis occurs.

185 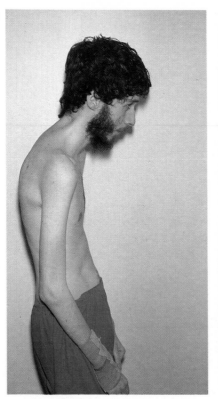 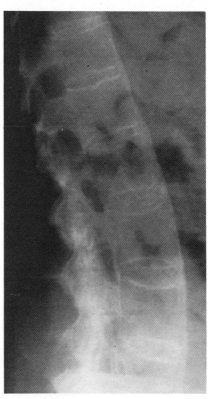 **186**

185 & 186 Advanced spinal AS. The posture may deteriorate seriously. In this patient the development of a severe and irreversible dorsal kyphosis is complicated by cervical spine stiffening, and he is beginning to experience difficulty seeing ahead. *This should be avoidable if treatment is initiated early and the patient cooperates with a regular exercise programme.* He breathes abdominally and the abdomen is typically protuberant. There is marked syndesmophyte formation on the lumbar spine X-ray (**186**). The patient also has severe peripheral joint involvement.

187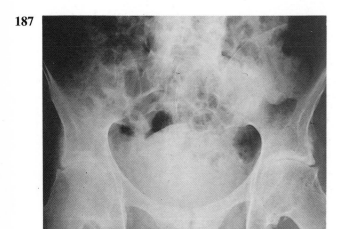

187 Pelvis with fused sacroiliac joints and severe hip disease. Peripheral joint involvement is usually part of an asymmetrical, pauciarticular (defined as affecting 2–4 joints) arthritis, predominantly of the large joints. This is the same patient as shown in **185 & 186**. Damage to the hip joint, which has greatly increased his disability, has worsened rapidly, leading to fixed flexion deformities of the hips and a further deterioration in posture. Despite the patient's youth, total hip replacement is the only realistic answer.

188 Spinal fusion due to calcification of the intervertebral ligaments in advanced AS. In addition to calcification of the intervertebral ligaments, fusion of the spinal facet joints and of the costovertebral joints may eventually lead to the clinical and radiological appearances of a so-called 'bamboo' spine. This patient, who already had a bamboo spine and had undergone bilateral hip replacements, developed diarrhoea. Because of the possibility of inflammatory bowel disease (*see* p.90), he underwent a barium enema, but no abnormality was demonstrated.

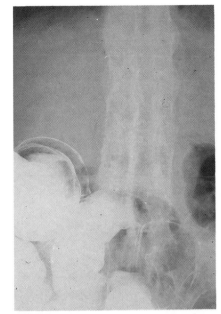

188

189

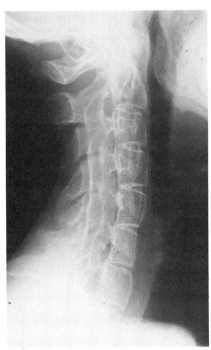

190

189 & 190 Cervical spine. This patient with juvenile onset disease has virtually complete spinal ankylosis. The posterior facet joints of the neck are fused in the earlier film (**189**). In the second film (**190**), taken seven years later, there is also complete calcification of the intervertebral ligaments and marked osteoporosis. In such cases, atlantoaxial instability may arise, the risk of which is increased by the fact that the patient's minimal residual head movement occurs at the atlantoaxial level. Regular neurological examination is indicated, and extra care should be exercised during intubation for anaesthesia (*see also* **68–78**). Spinal instability can develop at any nonankylosed level, especially where there is extensive spinal fusion both above and below that level, and may produce severe pain. Surgical fusion may be necessary. The abnormal lower cervical vertebral bodies reflect the fact that this patient's disease started in his early teens and led to bone-modelling abnormalities.

191

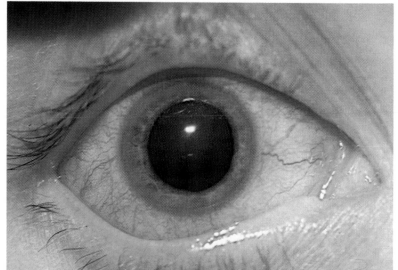

191 Acute anterior uveitis. The involvement of the uvea in individuals with AS and other seronegative spondarthritides is strongly associated with the presence of HLA B27. Uveitis can occur independently of the activity of the spinal disease and is sometimes the presenting feature, in which case a history of spinal stiffness and pain may be elicited upon careful questioning. The clinical symptoms of acute anterior uveitis are severe eye pain, photophobia and blurred vision. They are often so unbearable that the patient presents to a casualty department. Inflammation is worst around the periphery of the iris, producing circumcorneal injection, which is typically dusky purple. (In this picture the pupil is dilated therapeutically to prevent the development of posterior synechiae – *see* **193**).

192

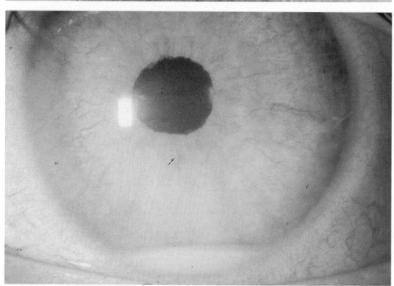

192 Acute anterior uveitis with hypopyon. In cases of very acute uveitis, an inflammatory exudate may be seen as a fluid level (hypopyon) in the anterior chamber, or as deposits (keratic precipitates) on the posterior surface of the cornea. The latter are best seen by slit-lamp examination. Urgent specialist advice should be sought if uveitis is suspected. Early topical treatment with corticosteroids (or occasionally with a subconjunctival injection) is essential. The pupil should be dilated until the attack has settled, both to relieve symptoms and to prevent adhesion of the iris to the lens (synechia). All patients at risk should be warned to report to a doctor immediately if eye pain and redness develop.

193

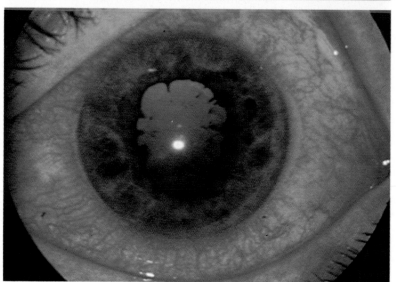

193 Posterior synechiae. The irregular appearance of the dilated pupil is due to the formation of adhesions between the iris and the anterior surface of the lens. Early treatment of acute attacks is essential if this is to be avoided. The development of glaucoma is a longer-term risk in such cases.

Management of AS

The key to effective management of AS is to engage the patient's enthusiasm for daily exercise, as a means of preventing long-term spinal stiffness and deformity. This requires careful explanation and regular encouragement: explanation of the importance of exercise during flares, when pain and stiffness are at their worst and tend to discourage movement; explanation of the need to take NSAIDs at night during such acute flares, primarily to control the early morning stiffness and pain so that the exercises are carried out fully and effectively; and encouragement to stop taking NSAIDs between flares, but nevertheless to continue with the daily exercise programme.

The exercises are best taught initially by a therapist. They involve a programme to put the whole spine through a full range of movements, to maintain normal posture and to encourage chest expansion. This approach will reduce the long-term risks of stiffness and deformity due to spinal fusion, and probably also reduces the risk of spinal osteoporosis. During acute flares, exercise in a warm-water pool is therapeutic and comforting. There is a wide network of self-help support groups for those with AS.

Patients should be warned of the risk of developing uveitis, and the importance of reporting any eye pain or redness promptly should be emphasised. If patients develop recurrent attacks, they will need regular ophthalmological review. In such cases it is often appropriate for them to initiate their own topical corticosteroid treatment as soon as eye pain develops.

Peripheral joint disease can be difficult to treat. Local flares are best dealt with by local corticosteroid injections. In more severe, polyarticular disease the use of sulphasalazine or, occasionally, of cytotoxic agents may be appropriate. External X-ray therapy was often used for spinal and, occasionally, for peripheral joint disease in the 1940s and 1950s. It is less frequently used now because, although it often produced excellent therapeutic responses, they were not always long-lived and there is a slight but definitely increased risk of developing local skin malignancies and leukaemia.

A few patients require surgery – either joint replacement or, occasionally, spinal osteotomy and/or fusion.

Diet may play a role if the faecal load of *Klebsiella* spp. is relevant, and some have advocated a diet that is low in carbohydrates.

Psoriatic arthritis

Table 12. Subtypes of psoriatic arthritis.

Distal interphalangeal joint arthritis (often with adjacent nail dystrophy)

Asymmetrical mono- or pauciarticular arthritis

Seronegative rheumatoid-like arthritis

Psoriatic arthritis mutilans

Psoriatic sacroiliitis/spondylitis (50% HLA B27 positive)

Common diseases such as seropositive RA and/or nodular OA may coexist with psoriasis

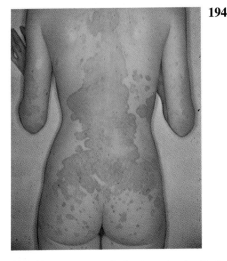

194

194 Cutaneous psoriasis. Associated with the possession of HLA B8, psoriasis is a common skin disease which affects up to 2% of the population. It presents as raised, red, nonitchy plaques, usually occurring over the extensor surfaces of the limbs, around the navel, in the natal cleft (a site in which it is often missed) or on the scalp. It may cause little trouble, but can be unsightly and extensive. It is sometimes life-threatening. About 8% of individuals with psoriasis develop one of a variety of articular complications. The skin disease and arthritis rarely correspond in terms of severity, usually flaring asynchronously.

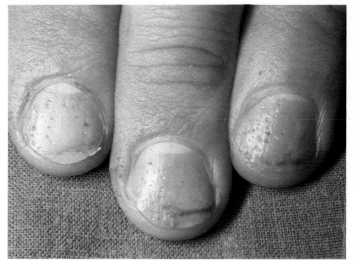

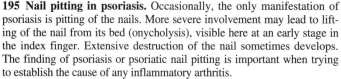

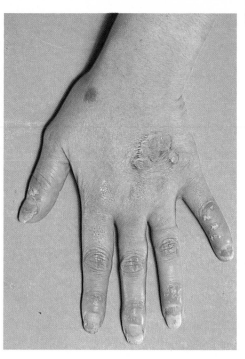

195 Nail pitting in psoriasis. Occasionally, the only manifestation of psoriasis is pitting of the nails. More severe involvement may lead to lifting of the nail from its bed (onycholysis), visible here at an early stage in the index finger. Extensive destruction of the nail sometimes develops. The finding of psoriasis or psoriatic nail pitting is important when trying to establish the cause of any inflammatory arthritis.

196 DIP joint involvement in psoriatic arthritis with severe nail dystrophy. In psoriatic arthritis, DIP joint involvement is the most typical and frequent pattern to be seen, with the joints becoming inflamed and swollen (*see* the IP joints of this patient's thumb and the DIP joint of the middle finger). A similar pattern may occur in the toes.

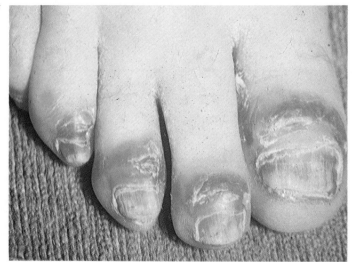

197 Nail dystrophy and DIP joint involvement. Toenail dystrophy has affected the great toe, which is also shortened by chronic IP joint damage. All of the toes show skin, nail and DIP involvement. A similar picture may develop, with or without skin changes, in Reiter's disease (*see* **205**)

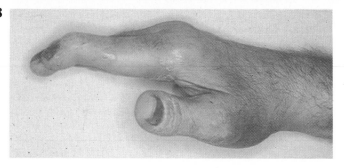

198 Rheumatoid-like seronegative arthritis with psoriasis. Sometimes, a more symmetrical arthritis may complicate psoriasis. It is rarely as destructive as severe RA, but may resemble it. Here, MCP synovitis and swan-necking of the PIP joints are associated with arthritis of the DIP joints.

199 Erosive arthropathy in psoriatic arthritis.
On this X-ray, damage to some of the joints mimics that seen in RA, with erosions and loss of joint space. In other joints the appearances are more typical of psoriatic arthritis (DIP joints of the right little finger and left ring finger, and MCP joint of the left little finger): symmetrical erosion of the distal end of the proximal bone and central erosion of the proximal end of the distal bone have produced what is sometimes called a 'pencil in cup' appearance. The IP joint of the left thumb is also extensively damaged and the wrists demonstrate early erosions and loss of joint space. The overall asymmetry and the DIP involvement suggest psoriatic arthritis. In contrast with RA, there is no female preponderance in this type of arthritis.

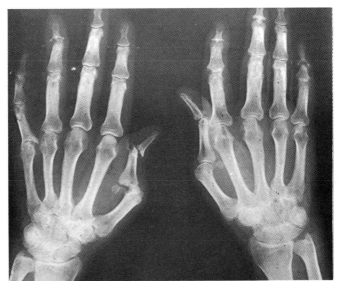

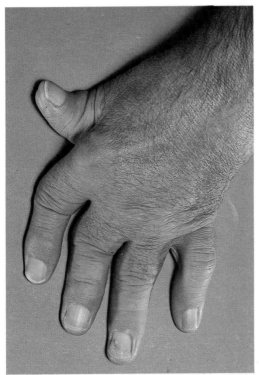

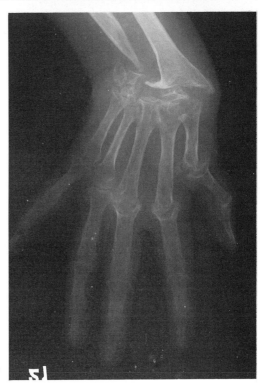

200 'Arthritis mutilans' in psoriatic arthritis.
Although a typical manifestation of psoriatic arthritis, arthritis mutilans is also its least common form, affecting about 5% of patients with articular disease. (A similar arthritis mutilans occasionally complicates seropositive RA). The erosion and eventual osteolysis of juxta-articular bone leads to shortening of the bones – so-called 'telescopic fingers'. Pain is not always severe and, despite the deformity, function is often reasonably retained. The joints are unstable and function may be improved by IP joint fusion (*see* **353**).

201 Arthritis mutilans. The destructive effects of the arthritis can be seen in this patient with a 7-year history. There are widespread erosions, and shortening due to osteolysis is apparent in the fifth proximal phalanx. This patient had a rheumatoid-like arthritis with mild psoriasis.

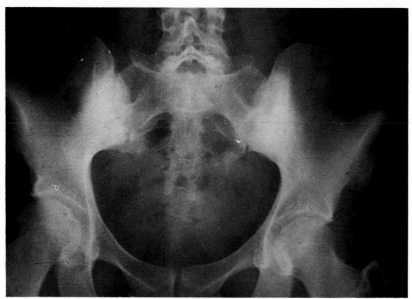

202 Psoriatic spondylitis. Individuals with psoriasis may also develop unilateral or, as here, bilateral sacroiliitis and, occasionally, spinal involvement similar to that seen in AS. In psoriatic spondylitis the neck may be affected before the thoracolumbar region, and the syndesmophytes may be less symmetrical than in typical AS. Once an infective cause has been excluded, unilateral sacroiliitis on X-ray is more-or-less diagnostic of psoriatic spondylitis. An association with HLA B27 does exist, but it is less significant than in AS; approximately 50% of patients with psoriasis and sacroiliitis are HLA B27-positive. The reason for this reduced positivity is not known, but it suggests that there may be other important aetiopathogenetic factors in this variant of AS.

Management of psoriatic arthritis

NSAIDs to control the pain and stiffness are the mainstay of management for patients, although the mildest cases may need no drug treatment at all. The pauciarticular pattern is best managed by local corticosteroid injections or, occasionally, by synovectomy. In the small proportion of cases that are severe, second-line drugs should be tried, along the lines suggested for RA (*see* p.48). (Antimalarials may worsen the skin disease and are best avoided.) Physiotherapy to maintain normal ranges of joint movement and mucle power is often helpful in the more severely affected cases.

Skin involvement may be mild and cause few skin problems. Sun exposure reduces the severity of the lesions. In moderate and severe cases, however, therapy may include locally applied coal tar derivatives and/or local corticosteroids. Courses of UV-A light, combined with oral psoralen, are sometimes used. In the most severe cases of skin disease, joint involvement (if present) may also be severe, and oral weekly methotrexate is the treatment of choice; monitoring of full blood count and liver and lung function are obligatory (*see* p.48).

Nail dystrophy is best managed with topical corticosteroids, but can prove resistant.

Reactive arthritis (Reiter's disease)

The classic triad of signs in Reiter's disease comprises **acute asymmetrical lower limb arthritis**, a **nonspecific urethritis** (NSU) and **mild conjunctivitis**. 'Incomplete' cases occur, in which conjunctivitis is absent or so mild that it is not complained of. The arthritis, which occurs more commonly in males, develops a few days to a couple of weeks after an attack of NSU. In the male, NSU usually presents to a genitourinary medicine department with dysuria, and a purulent penile discharge, although it is occasionally asymptomatic or unnoticed. Nonspecific cervicitis in the female is usually asymptomatic and is easily missed without a careful examination. With the third problem of the triad, the conjunctiva is injected, feels gritty and there is crusting of the eyes in the morning. Reactive arthritis complicating asymptomatic nonspecific cervicitis may account for otherwise unexplained lower limb arthritis in the female. Treatment of NSU with tetracyclines does not affect the course of the arthritis. Coexistent gonorrhoea and other sexually transmitted diseases need exclusion, and referral to a specialist genitourinary medicine department is essential.

In Europe, reactive arthritis now more commonly follows a bout of **bacillary dysentery** (due to *Salmonella* or *Shigella* spp.) or of **diarrhoea** due to infection with the micro-organism *Yersinia enterocolitica*.

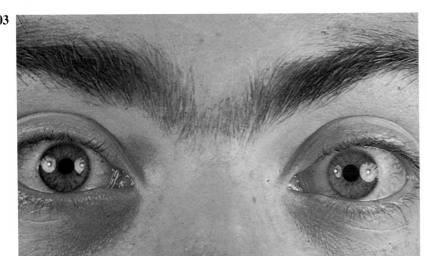

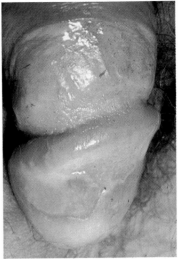

203 Conjunctivitis in a man with acute monarthritis and NSU. The conjunctivitis of reactive arthritis is almost always bilateral, unlike the more common viral conjunctivitis. It may be mild and overlooked by patients, especially as the joint or genital disease or the diarrhoea is often more worrying. In a proportion of patients no history of eye involvement is obtained; this is sometimes called incomplete Reiter's syndrome. Acute anterior uveitis (*see* 191) is unusual in the early stages of the disease, but it may complicate the more severe or relapsing case and should not be missed. Patients are best warned to report urgently any undue eye pain.

204 Circinate balanitis. In the uncircumcised male the glans penis may develop painless, superficial, ulcerative lesions. These cause alarm, but heal without scarring. In the circumcised male the lesion tends to be raised, reddened and scaly, mimicking psoriatic lesions. The problem (as with the joint disease) can recur and, as long as genital reinfection has not occurred, is not itself contagious. Similar ulcerative lesions sometimes arise around the penile meatus, and on the cervix in the female. Aphthous ulceration of the mouth may also occur.

205 Keratoderma blennorrhagica. As shown here, the cutaneous lesions of patients with reactive arthritis occur typically on the feet as painless, reddened, often confluent, raised plaques and pustules. They are similar, both clinically and histologically, to the lesions of pustular psoriasis. Nail dystrophy may also occur, as here. These similarities underline the overlap between the seronegative spondarthritides. There is marked inflammation of the toe joints of the left foot, and destructive changes have led to shortening of the left great toe.

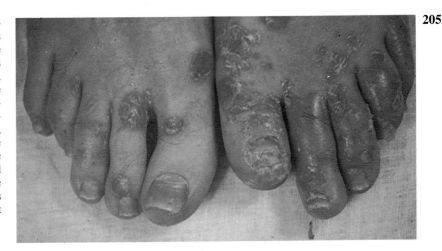

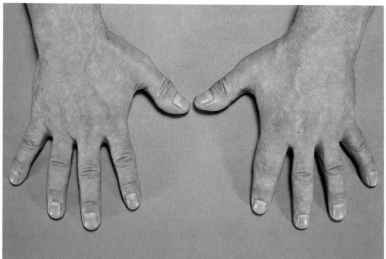

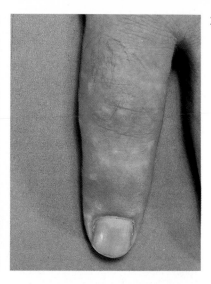

206 & 207 Dactylitis in postdysenteric Reiter's disease. This patient had developed dysentery 3 weeks before he presented, complaining of swollen knees, a swollen ankle and a stiff, swollen left index finger. Synovitis of the DIP, PIP and MCP joints was found, in addition to flexor tenosynovitis and an effusion in the tendon sheath. He responded well to a local steroid injection into the tendon sheath, together with a 4-week course of NSAIDs.

208

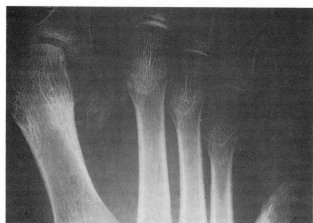

208 Periostitis in recurrent reactive arthritis. The majority of patients with reactive arthritis experience an initial attack of arthritis which settles. Some, however, progress to a more chronic relapsing and remitting form, which can be highly disabling. Certain individuals develop periostitis, which can here be seen affecting the distal cortex of the fifth metatarsal. The reason for this type of periosteal reaction is not clear, but it is unusual in other forms of inflammatory arthritis. Erosive changes involving the adjacent fifth MTP joint are also apparent.

In susceptible individuals with reactive arthritis, sacroiliitis and spondylitis may also develop.

209

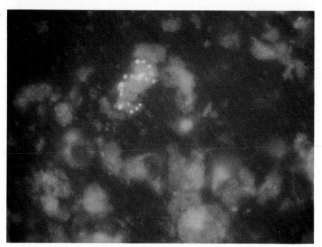

209 Chlamydial 'primary bodies', demonstrated by immunostaining in the joint effusion of a patient with reactive arthritis. In about 50% of patients, *Chlamydia* or *Ureaplasma* can be cultured from the urethra, and/or a rising titre of specific antibodies is detected in the blood. The most exciting recent development has been the detection of lipopolysaccharides derived from *Chlamydia* and other relevant organisms in the inflamed synovium of affected joints. These particles, here seen in the cellular deposit from a sample of synovial fluid, are not infective, but they indicate that the inflammatory reaction may be triggered locally by micro-organisms or their derivatives, rather than being a distant immunological reaction to infection at other sites (compare poststreptococcal arthritis, p.120).

210 & 211 Painful heel in reactive arthritis. Heel pain is a common feature of reactive arthritis and may be due to an inflammatory lesion at the insertion of the plantar fascia into the calcaneum. This produces localised tenderness under the heel, with pain on weight-bearing. This may warrant treatment by a local corticosteroid injection (*see* p.154). In some patients a lesion at the insertion of the Achilles tendon causes posterior heel pain when walking. The discomfort is worse during the heel-lift phase and when walking barefoot; a shoe with a heel and an additional heel pad decreases the tension in the Achilles tendon, thereby reducing the pain. The radiological appearance seen in **210** is of calcaneal spurs which have poorly defined outlines (in contrast with the sharp, beak-like outline of the so-called degenerative spur in **211**). Erosions may also develop at the upper pole of the calcaneum, near the insertion of the Achilles tendon.

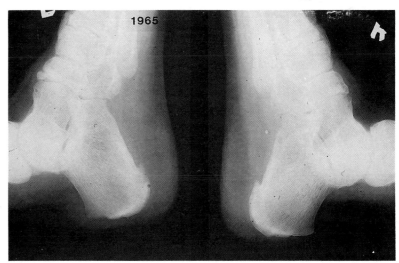

210

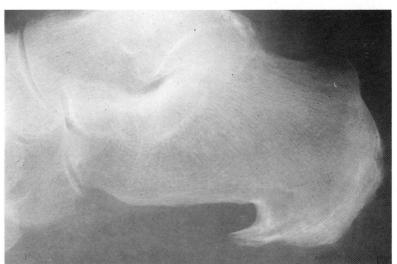

211

Management of reactive arthritis

Although antibiotic treatment of the precipitating infection is sometimes undertaken, there is little evidence that it significantly affects the long-term outcome of reactive arthritis when it develops in susceptible individuals. This may be partly due to the fact that the triggering of the reactive arthritis occurs early in the infection, before symptoms are troublesome. Indeed, for many it is the joint disease, rather than the infection, which first precipitates a medical consultation.

Specialist advice should be sought to detect and treat any coexisting sexually transmitted diseases when the arthritis has been precipitated by NSU or cervicitis. It should be borne in mind that reactive arthritis (with or without cutaneous psoriasiform lesions) may, rarely, be the first presentation of AIDS (*see* p.126).

For most patients, reactive arthritis is transient and can be managed with NSAIDs. Not infrequently, a joint may be greatly swollen, warranting aspiration and a corticosteroid injection. In the relapsing case, intermittent courses of NSAIDs may be sufficient, but others may require sulphasalazine or another second-line drug (*see* p.48). In such cases the involvement of a physiotherapist is essential and, occasionally, surgical intervention is necessary.

Enteropathic arthritis of Crohn's disease and ulcerative colitis

An asymmetrical, predominantly lower limb arthritis which is independent of possession of the HLA B27 antigen and/or an HLA B27 associated sacroiliitis or spondylitis may be seen in about 5% of individuals with either Crohn's disease or ulcerative colitis. In some instances, the rheumatological symptoms may predate the development of the bowel disease or lead to its diagnosis. The creation of a blind loop by intestinal bypass surgery for morbid obesity is occasionally associated with a similar arthritis: this procedure is no longer performed so commonly because of the risk of hepatic complications. The link between the bowel and arthritis is now widely recognised, although it is still poorly understood. The possibility that selective mucosal leakiness to pathogens or antigens may lead to joint disease remains fascinating but unproven.

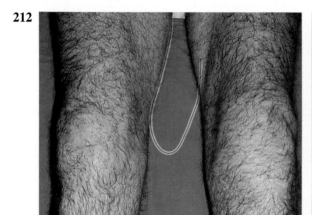

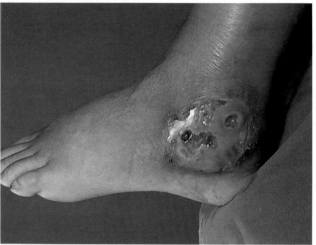

212 Acute monarthritis of the knee in a patient with Crohn's disease. This man first presented with a monarthritis of the knee. He suffered recurrent arthritis of the knees and ankles over several years, before eventually developing rectal bleeding. A colonic biopsy revealed the typical granulomatous changes of Crohn's disease. His father had Reiter's disease and his sister developed Crohn's disease without joint involvement.

213 Pyoderma gangrenosum complicating ulcerative colitis. This young woman presented with a swollen elbow and bloody diarrhoea. A reactive arthritis was initially suspected, although no organism was cultured from the stools. She later developed an acutely painful swelling around the lateral malleolus. The overlying skin broke, discharging sterile pus. The histology was typical of pyoderma gangrenosum and the patient made a full recovery with a course of oral corticosteroids. Pyoderma gangrenosum is an unusual complication of inflammatory bowel disease; colonic biopsy in this patient later revealed typical ulcerative colitis to be the cause of the diarrhoea. Erythema nodosum (*see* **305**) may also complicate ulcerative colitis.

Management of enteropathic arthritis

Remission of any associated joint disease usually accompanies remission of ulcerative colitis or total colectomy, and reversal of a surgically-induced intestinal bypass is curative of any associated joint disease. However, arthritis settles less frequently in Crohn's disease, even after effective treatment of the bowel. In all cases of enteropathic arthritis the joint disease should be managed symptomatically with NSAIDs. A monarthritis is best treated with intra-articular corticosteroids. Sulphasalazine is frequently prescribed and appears to help both the bowel and the joint disease. Sacroiliitis or spondylitis may be asymptomatic, but the management is the same as that for AS (*see* p.83). Patients with spondylitis rarely remit fully, even if the associated bowel disease can be controlled.

7 Other autoimmune connective tissue disorders

Autoimmune connective tissue disorders comprise a wide spectrum of systemic diseases of unknown aetiology. All of the disorders are relatively uncommon, but important to recognise and treat. Although they exhibit a variety of clinical features, they are unified by the presence of nonorgan-specific autoantibodies, found in the serum and in various tissues. The cells and the extracellular matrix of the connective tissues are invariably affected, although this is not unique to this group of diseases. The mechanisms of damage are ill-understood. Occasionally, the typical features of two or more disorders may coexist in the same patient – an 'overlap' syndrome. Individuals with autoimmune connective tissue disorders are difficult to manage and require careful monitoring. It is in the interest both of the patients and of further research that they are cared for by specialist units.

Table 13. Non organ-specific autoantibodies.

Rheumatoid factors	Antibodies for which the Fc portion of immunoglobulin is the antigen (*see* p.15). Detected routinely in the IgM form, but also present as IgG and IgA RF. Detected in, but not diagnostic of RA – a high titre indicates a worse prognosis. Positive titres may predate the onset of RA. They are also present at varying frequencies in most other autoimmune rheumatic disorders and many chronic infections, appearing in low titres in asymptomatic older individuals.
Antinuclear antibodies	ANAs are detected in a wide variety of autoimmune diseases. They are an important first screening test for SLE, but are nonspecific, as low titres may be detectable in infections and some neoplastic diseases. The pattern of fluorescent staining on fresh–frozen sections of rodent liver or rabbit kidney, or Hep-2 cell lines reflects differing antigenic specificities, which are associated with different clinical conditions. For example, a nucleolar or an anticentromere pattern is usually found in scleroderma, whereas a homogeneous pattern with or without rim enhancement is typical of anti-DNA/histone antibodies found in lupus.
Anti-double-stranded-DNA antibodies	The detection of antibodies against double-stranded DNA is important in the diagnosis of SLE (although patients with mild or inactive disease may be negative). High titres of the IgG isotype often indicate a poor prognosis and are not found in other diseases. (Anti-single-stranded DNA antibodies are much less specific.)
Anti-RNA antibodies	Although some groups have reported these antibodies to be confined to lupus patients, others have described them in a range of autoimmune rheumatic diseases.
Anti-extractable-nuclear-antigen (ENA) antibodies	These antibodies produce a speckled ANA fluorescent pattern. Generally included are antibodies to Ro, La, Sm and RNP, although other antigens have been identified in similar cell extracts. Anti-La is strongly associated with Sjögren's syndrome, anti-Ro with SLE/Sjögren's and anti-Sm with SLE. Anti-RNP antibodies are found in a range of diseases including SLE, and were once thought to be diagnostic of mixed connective tissue disorder (MCTD), but this is now thought to be a dubious disease entity.
Anti-neutrophil-cytoplasmic-antibodies (ANCA)	These are found in most cases of systemic vasculitis, particularly, but not exclusively, in Wegener's granulomatosis. They produce either perinuclear or granular staining patterns.

Systemic lupus erythematosus

Systemic lupus erythematosus (SLE) has an extremely wide range of clinical manifestations, varying from the mild to the potentially fatal. It often presents in young women, with protean features; most commonly fever, malaise, arthritis and a rash arise, but any manifestation may exist separately. A great mimic of other diseases, SLE can prove difficult to diagnose. It should be included in the differential diagnosis of a pyrexia of unknown origin. Raynaud's phenomenon (*see* **218**), photosensitivity, alopecia, pleurisy, mouth ulceration, headaches, convulsions, acute psychosis and acute glomerulonephritis may all occur. The first episode, or subsequent flares, may be precipitated by excessive exposure to ultraviolet light, by pregnancy, or after starting the contraceptive pill or hormone replacement therapy. Renal involvement, particularly in the form of a proliferative glomerulonephritis or the nephrotic syndrome, and cerebral involvement are both poor prognostic indicators and are potentially fatal unless immediate therapy is instituted. Antinuclear antibodies (ANAs) are not diagnostic as they occur in other diseases, but they are present in 90% of patients with SLE. Antibodies to double-stranded DNA are more disease-specific, but occur at some time in only 75% of affected patients; they usually signify more severe disease (*see* **Table 13**). The ANAs form immune complexes in the circulation and tissues, and it is these complexes that are the probable triggers of the immunologically induced tissue damage.

A variety of drugs, including hydralazine, methyldopa, isoniazid and D-penicillamine, can induce antinuclear antibodies in susceptible individuals, but not antibodies to double-stranded DNA. Only a small number of individuals, however, develops a lupus-like disease, which is generally mild and reverses when the drug is discontinued.

214

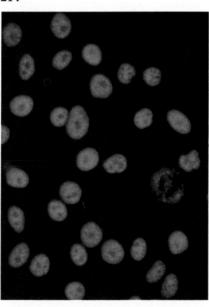

214 Immunofluorescence of ANAs. ANAs are not species-specific and are detected by using thin slices of rat liver or rabbit kidney as the substrate. The bound antibodies are then visualised by binding to fluorescein-labelled antihuman antibodies and viewed under ultraviolet light. Different patterns of staining indicate different intranuclear (or cytoplasmic) antigens (*see* **Table 13**). The staining of the nucleus may be homogeneous, with or without other superimposed patterns. The peripheral (rim-enhanced) pattern correlates to anti-dsDNA antibodies. A speckled pattern (shown here) may occur in SLE, but it is more common in scleroderma and Sjögren's disease. Nucleolar or anticentromere staining is usually found in scleroderma. The 'LE cell' test is much less specific and clincally outdated, although it is still of historical interest.

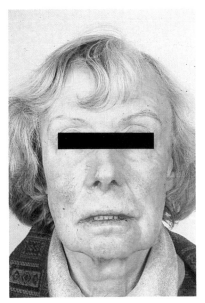 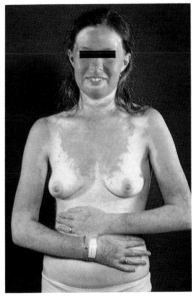

215 & 216 Typical light-sensitive rash in SLE. Although it is not the only skin manifestation, the so-called 'butterfly rash' which sometimes occurs over the bridge of the nose and the upper cheeks illustrates the role of ultraviolet (UV) light in inducing skin damage in SLE. The forehead, lips and chin are also affected. The patient in **216** had recently returned from a seaside holiday and demonstrates a more striking photosensitivity reaction than that shown in **215**. A wide variety of other cutaneous manifestations may occur in SLE, and drug sensitivity rashes are common.

217 Normal hand X-ray in long-standing SLE with persistent arthralgia. This patient experienced severe joint pain for several years without much clinical evidence of synovitis and without developing radiological damage. Complaints of pain that is apparently out of proportion to the clinical joint involvement are typical of SLE. Indeed, unless this is borne in mind, the disease may be missed if such pain is the main complaint. It is not uncommon for affected patients to be labelled as 'hysterical'. Occasionally, an erosive arthritis does occur, reflecting an overlap with RA; very rarely, ulnar deviation also develops, without radiological evidence of joint damage. This resembles the now rare nonerosive deforming arthritis of the hands, first described by Jaccoud in severe, recurrent rheumatic fever (*see* p.120). It is caused by weakening of the MCP joint capsules and their associated tendon attachments (due to local inflammation).

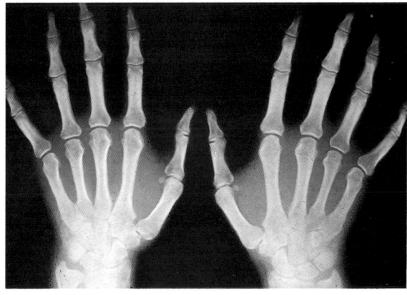

217

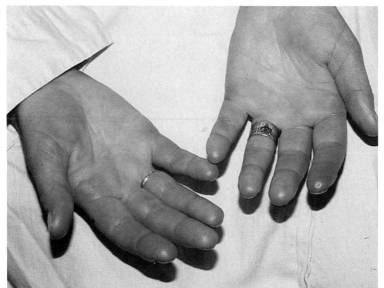

218 Raynaud's phenomenon. Raynaud's phenomenon is a vasospastic disorder with a typical triphasic colour response to cold. After initial pallor, the fingers (rarely the toes or nose) turn absolutely white. There is then a brief period of cyanosis (illustrated here), followed by painful redness due to rebound hyperaemia. The phenomenon is not specific to SLE and may arise in any of the connective tissue disorders, particularly scleroderma (*see* p.97), and in RA. In young women a similar phenomenon may occur in isolation. It has also been reported as an industrial disease in men who use pneumatic drills or other vibrating tools. Should it arise *de novo*, particularly in an older woman, or a man at any age, and especially if complicated by digital ulceration, an underlying systemic disease must always be considered. Most cases are managed by avoidance of extreme cold or sudden changes of temperature, but vasodilator drugs such as nifedipine may be required by some patients.

219 & 220 Acute proliferative glomerulonephritis. Any patient with SLE should be checked regularly for renal involvement, especially early in the disease. Blood pressure must be measured at each visit, and fresh urine tested for blood and/or protein. If either proteinuria or haematuria is detected, the urinary sediment should be examined for cells or casts, and a 24-hour urine collection checked for total protein excretion and creatinine clearance. A wide variety of different histological pictures may be seen. **219** shows subendothelial deposits ('wire loops') stained as bright red chunks with Masson's trichrome. **220** demonstrates a silver stain: the changes revealed are more chronic, with mesangial deposits as well as subendothelial deposits. Urgent specialist advice is required. Although some renal appearances are relatively benign, others require high doses of steroids and cytotoxic agents – steroids alone are usually insufficient. Correctly and quickly managed, the outlook is no longer as serious as was the case only a few years ago.

221 Brain scan demonstrating cerebral vasculitis. There is dispute about the significance and frequency of neuropsychiatric problems in SLE, although mild abnormalities are detectable in many patients upon careful psychometric testing. The most important cerebral complications arise from a focal or generalised cerebral vasculitis, which can be demonstrated by isotope brain scanning, CT or, as shown here, by MRI. There are small foci of high signal in the frontal and parietal white matter (arrows). The appearances are not specific, reflecting ischaemic lesions which may also arise from hypertensive disease, for example.

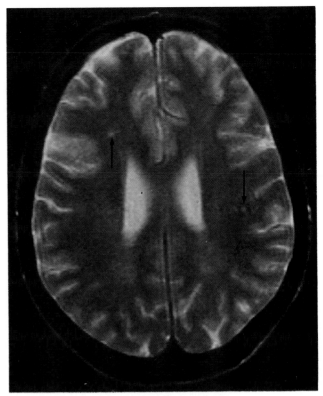

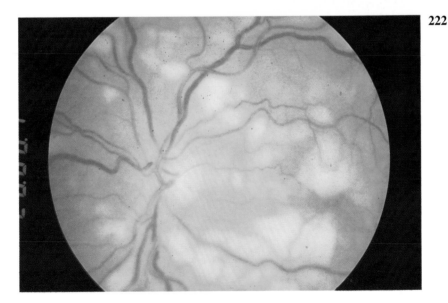

222 SLE retinopathy. Retinal vessels occasionally allow direct visualisation of vasculopathies. This picture is a colour retinal photograph showing multiple, coalescent cotton-wool spots and retinal vasculitis. This type of retinal ischaemic picture may be seen in SLE. Fluorescein angiography can often demonstrate more subtle abnormalities earlier. Leakage of the dye indicates areas of active vasculitis. Complete blockage of vessels may be demonstrated in either the arterial or venous phase pictures.

223

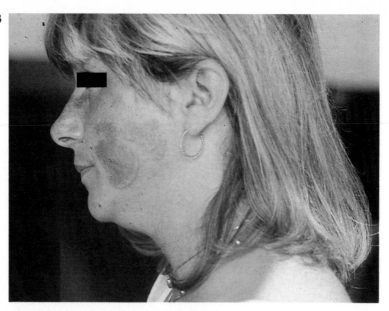

223 & 224 Discoid lupus – lupus band test. Discoid lupus is a well-demarcated chronic skin rash which is usually confined to the head, arms or upper trunk. There is prominent scaling, keratotic plugging, atrophy and telangiectasia. Alopecia is invariable in hairy areas. There is permanent scarring. Only a small proportion of patients with discoid lupus goes on to develop SLE. A biopsy of the lesion itself will reveal the deposition of immunoglobulin and complement (a lupus band) at the dermoepidermal junction (**224**), but unaffected skin will be normal.

A positive lupus band in unaffected skin indicates systemic lupus and is a helpful diagnostic test.

224

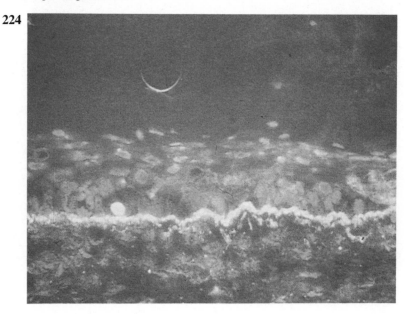

Management of SLE

Patients are often aware of the poor outlook for some, but not the majority of cases of SLE. Careful counselling and psychological support may be necessary to reduce inappropriate anxiety.

A variety of drugs can be used, according to the symptoms and the severity of the disease. It is clear that one of the reasons for the overall improvement in the outlook of SLE in recent years has been a more cautious and appropriate use of the more toxic drugs, under the supervision of specialist clinics. Another factor is apparent rather than actual, and reflects the fact that milder cases, with a better prognosis, are now being recognised with the help of more accurate tests for antinuclear antibodies.

Arthralgia (which may be severe), arthritis, fever and serositis respond to NSAIDs, which are usually the only drugs needed in the milder forms of the disease.

Antimalarial drugs (chloroquine or hydroxy-chloroquine) in low doses help the same spectrum of symptoms as the NSAIDs, together with milder cutaneous involvement, and may be used in combination with them. Initial and regular ophthalmological studies are obligatory to detect any retinal damage caused by antimalarials, although this is rare with the low doses now used. Hydroxychloroquine is more expensive, but it is probably less likely to produce retinal problems.

If these milder symptoms are still not satisfactorily controlled, or if more serious disease occurs (i.e., renal involvement, vasculitis, blood dyscrasias or cerebral disease) corticosteroids in low oral doses or by intravenous bolus delivery, and/or cytotoxic drugs such as azathioprine or cyclophosphamide may be needed. All such cases require specialist supervision and careful monitoring.

Scleroderma, the CREST syndrome and systemic sclerosis

Scleroderma, the CREST sydrome and systemic sclerosis are rare diseases, the cardinal features of which are thickening and induration of the skin. There are associated abnormalities of small blood vessels, which can easily be seen in the nail fold, using a hand lens. Widespread telangiectasia may also arise. These vascular abnormalities may be the primary aetiological event. Raynaud's phenomenon is present in 90% of patients and is often severe. At a later stage, fibrosis of the skin and internal organs may develop. There is a wide spectrum of clinical disease. It may be apparently localised to the skin, either in patches (morphoea) or simply affecting the fingers and hands (sclerodactyly). One syndrome, usually known by the acronym 'CREST' (Calcinosis, Raynaud's phenomenon, oEsophageal involvement with reflux, Sclerodactyly and Telangiectasia), generally progresses slowly, but occasionally has a poor long-term outcome. Finally, there is the more diffuse disease, best called systemic sclerosis, which produces more serious systemic disease. This has a generally worse outlook and a significant mortality. All of the diseases are more common in women than in men, usually presenting in 30–50-year-olds. They are extremely rare in childhood.

Pathologically, deposition of collagen (particularly types I and III) in the skin and internal organs increases, fibroblast activity intensifies, and the collagen appears to be more difficult to break down. The trigger for this is unknown. A nucleolar or anticentromere staining pattern of ANA is usually found (*see* **Table 13**). Other ANAs may also be detected, as may rheumatoid factors.

A clinically similar picture may develop following industrial exposure to the solvent vinyl chloride. In a scandal in Spain in the 1980s, cooking oil was contaminated with rape seed oil, producing a severe illness in some of those exposed, again with some features of systemic sclerosis. In these cases the antinucleolar and anticentromere antibodies, which are relatively specific for the idiopathic systemic disease, were not found.

The classification of these diseases is complicated by the fact that some features may overlap with those of SLE, dermatomyositis or rheumatoid arthritis. There is also an association with Sjögren's syndrome (*see* **98–100** and p.108).

225

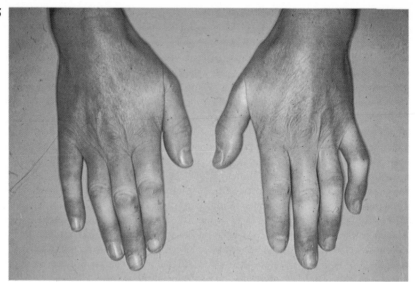

225 Early scleroderma. Raynaud's phenomenon (*see* **218**) develops in 90% of patients, often predating the onset of other symptoms and signs. Early scleroderma may produce diffuse swelling and stiffness of the fingers, which can resemble early RA, but there is a slow progression to waxy thickening and tethering of the skin over the fingers. These changes sometimes extend to the forearms and may affect the face and, occasionally, the trunk. In this patient, there is slight fixed flexion of the fingers. When an attempt is made to force them flat onto the desk, typical blanching around the knuckles develops.

226

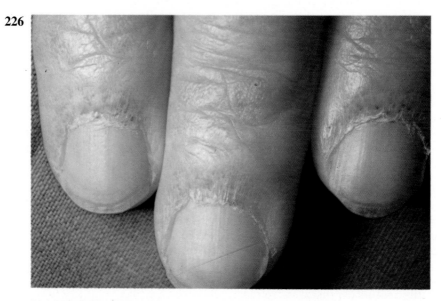

226 Nail fold capillary changes in scleroderma. In early disease these typical changes, which may be seen with a hand lens, are helpful in distinguishing scleroderma from RA. There is blunting of the normal capillary loops, striking capillary enlargement and relative loss of capillaries in adjacent areas. The cuticle is often ragged. Similar changes are seen in dermatomyositis (*see* **243**).

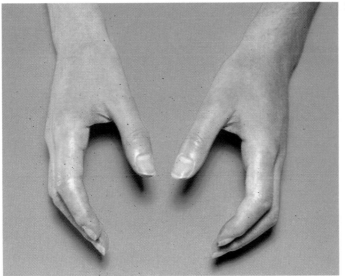

227 Advanced scleroderma. The hand involvement may progress to produce severe fixed flexion deformities of the fingers.

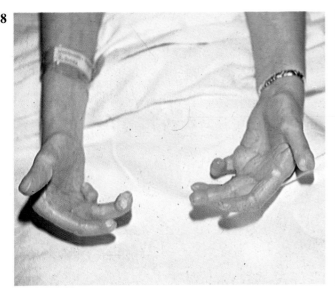

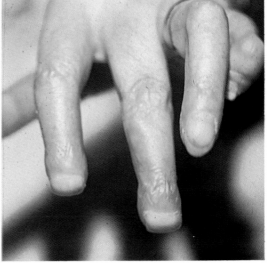

228 & 229 Scleroderma with calcinosis. Repeated and severe attacks of Raynaud's phenomenon lead to ulceration of the finger tips and, eventually, to loss of the finger pads. Gangrene of the fingers and/or toes may also occur. White deposits of calcinosis can be seen on the hands in both patients.

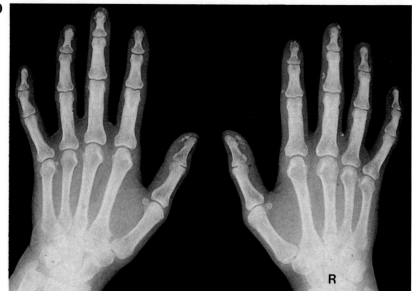

230 Radiology of the hand in scleroderma. This patient demonstrates the typical densely radio-opaque flecks of soft tissue calcinosis, best seen in the pulps of both thumbs and in the right middle finger. Necrosis of the finger pulp of the right index finger is also apparent.

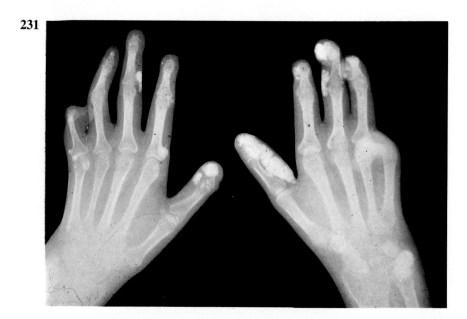

231 Radiology of the hand in advanced scleroderma. Gross deformities, with loss of the terminal phalanges and widespread large calcinotic deposits, can be seen in these hands. The patient is disabled by severe limitation of manual dexterity.

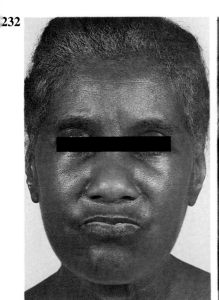

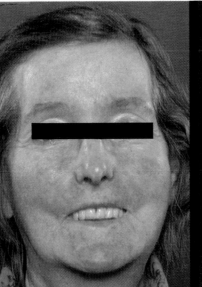

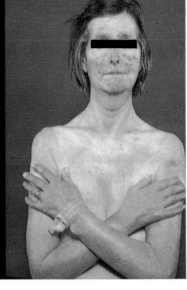

232 Facial scleroderma. Involvement of the facial skin leads to a pinched mouth and a taut expression. The normal skin folds are lost and may be replaced by radial lines running away from the mouth. Patients experience difficulty opening the mouth, which can lead to problems with eating and at the dentist.

233 Scleroderma with telangiectasia. Widespread facial telangiectasia has developed in this woman, together with facial and truncal skin involvement with scleroderma, which has led to thickened, fixed and shiny skin.

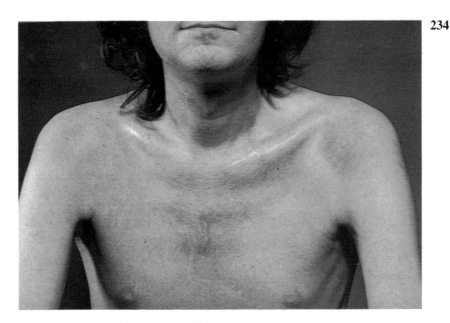

234 Severe truncal scleroderma. This male patient demonstrates the thickened and shiny skin of extensive cutaneous involvement, which may lead to marked restriction of chest expansion and a sense of the body being encased. Patchy hyperpigmentation and depigmentation of the skin may occur in cases of all types, from mild to severe.

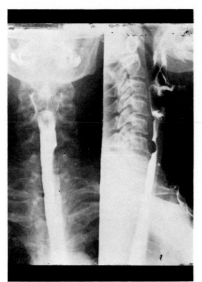

235 Oesophageal involvement in the CREST syndrome. The oesophagus may be affected, with neural plexus damage and muscular atrophy leading to abnormal neuromuscular coordination and, later, to dilatation of the oesophagus. The patient complains of heartburn, reflux or difficulty swallowing. A barium swallow demonstrates uncoordinated peristalsis when screened. Later in the disease, there may be oesophageal stricture formation which, together with dilatation of the atrophied muscular wall, increases the risk of overflow pneumonia from an oesophageal 'sump'. Small bowel involvement may also occur, resulting in dilated loops of bowel and malabsorption.

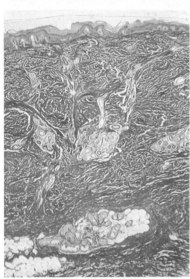

236 Skin histology of scleroderma. Extensive deposition of collagen throughout the dermis has extended into the subdermis. The epidermis is thin and atrophic, and the rete pegs no longer extend into the dermis. Adnexal structures, such as hair follicles and sweat glands, atrophy and may eventually disappear.

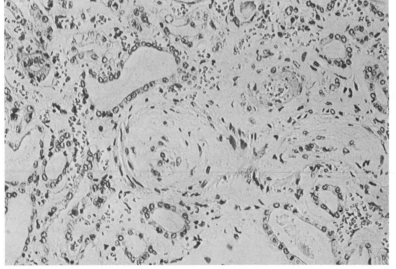

237 Renal involvement in systemic sclerosis. Renal involvement is the most common cause of death in systemic sclerosis. The use of angiotensin II-converting-enzyme (ACE) inhibitors and other antihypertensive agents has improved the prognosis significantly by controlling otherwise fatal malignant hypertension and averting the development of acute renal failure. Nevertheless the outlook for patients with renal disease is generally poor. Regular checks of blood pressure, along with urine examination for protein, cells or casts, are obligatory. On renal biopsy, there are abnormalities of cortical blood vessels, thrombotic occlusion of small arteries and focal glomerular changes. With time, interstitial fibrosis develops.

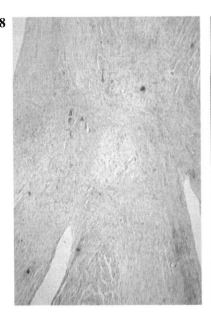
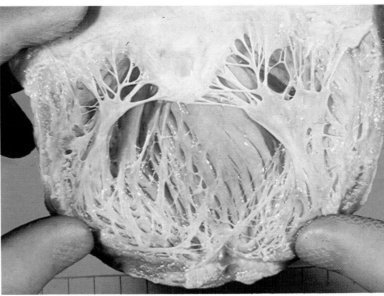

238 & 239 Cardiac fibrosis in systemic sclerosis. In severe cases, there is extensive abnormal collagen deposition in many organs. The lungs may become fibrotic and this, together with recurrent pneumonia due to overflow from the oesophagus, can be fatal. Regular testing of lung function is important. Cardiac involvement is frequently subclinical, but extensive fibrosis of the cardiac wall (seen here both microscopically and macroscopically) may lead to cardiac dysrhythmias, cardiomyopathy with severe congestive cardiac failure, or sudden death.

Management of scleroderma, the CREST syndrome and systemic sclerosis

Cases of scleroderma,the CREST syndrome and systemic sclerosis may, rarely, remit spontaneously, but generally require specialist management. Counselling and psychological support are important.

For Raynaud's phenomenon, avoidance of exposure to cold is essential, and electrically heated gloves and shoes may be indicated in severe cases. Patients should also refrain from smoking. In more severe cases, vasodilators such as nifedipine may help, as may cautious intermittent infusion of prostacyclin. The skin should be kept moist and any ulceration dressed carefully. Stiff hands may be helped by physiotherapy. There is, to date, no clearly effective way of con-trolling the fibrosis, although D-penicillamine or colchicine are sometimes tried. Corticosteroids may help in the early, oedematous phase or where there is muscle involvement, but the long-term benefit is unclear and they are probably best avoided.

Pulmonary disease may be helped by cortico-steroids in the early stages and antibiotics should be used if bronchitis or pneumonia develop. The outlook for established lung disease is poor.

Renal involvement is best treated by using ACE inhibitors and other antihypertensives, but the prognosis is again poor. Any heart failure should be treated appropriately.

Polymyositis and dermatomyositis

Polymyositis and dermatomyositis are best regarded as a group of rare disorders of unknown cause, in which the clinical picture is dominated by a nonsuppurative inflammation of striated muscle. Muscular involvement presents as proximal muscle weakness, initially of the legs, and patients experience difficulty squatting and getting up from a low chair. Later, the arms are affected and raising the hands above the head becomes difficult. More generalised muscle weakness may ensue. In severe cases, the muscles of respiration are involved and artificial ventilation may be required. Weakness is, however, of variable severity. In the acute phase, there is often general malaise, weight loss and fever. Leucocytosis and a raised ESR occur in about 50% of patients. Onset may be acute or insidious. The muscles are tender, but the patient generally complains of a combination of weakness and pain. This contrasts both with polymyalgia rheumatica (*see* p.135), in which stiffness and pain are the main complaints, and with myopathies, in which weakness is predominant, but not associated with pain or stiffness. Cutaneous involvement is common in childhood-onset disease, and is the dominant feature at presentation in about 25% of adult cases. These latter cases are referred to as dermatomyositis.

The definitive test to establish a diagnosis of polymyositis is a fine-needle muscle biopsy (usually of the quadriceps). In experienced hands this is quick, safe and painless (although the patient's clotting status should always be checked beforehand). The biopsy is not always positive, however, because of the patchy nature of the involvement (*see* **240–242**). The serum level of creatine phosphokinase (CPK) (predominantly the fraction derived from skeletal muscle) may be greatly raised in active polymyositis, but a normal result does not rule out the diagnosis. Electromyographic (EMG) changes may also be detected. The typical triad of changes comprises spontaneous fibrillation potentials at complete rest, polyphasic or short-duration potentials during voluntary contractions, and salvos of repetitive potentials on mechanical stimulation of the nerve. Only if the CPK, EMG and muscle biopsy are all normal can polymyositis be eliminated, and any one may be the only positive and diagnostic finding.

The cause of the disease is unknown, although in some it may be precipitated by exposure to light or by a viral illness. There is an association with HLA B8 and HLA DR3, suggesting an immunogenetic component. A variety of autoantibodies may be found. An antibody to the enzyme histidyl-tRNA synthetase, known as anti-Jo-1, is perhaps the most specific.

In adults (more commonly in males) polymyositis or dermatomyositis may be associated with a carcinoma of the lung, breast, female genitalia, prostate or bowel. Therefore, initial investigations should include a full clinical examination and a chest X-ray. More extensive tests for malignancy may be indicated, although opinions differ as to how necessary these are. Long-term follow-up is essential.

In untreated disease, and when treatment fails, the end result is often severe muscle fibrosis; there is a high risk of flexion contractures developing. Cutaneous scarring may be severe, especially in childhood disease, when extensive subcutaneous and myofascial calcinosis may also develop.

Overlap syndromes with scleroderma, SLE and RA can occur.

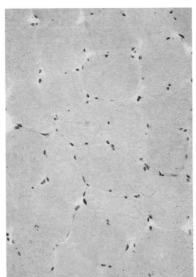

240–242 Muscle changes in polymyositis. The hallmark of biopsy appearances in polymyositis is the presence of an extensive inflammatory infiltrate around blood vessels and between the muscle fibres. The fibres demonstrate gross differences in diameter and size, reflecting both their degeneration and abnormal regeneration. Many fibres are necrotic. Normally, the nuclei of skeletal muscle lie peripherally in the fibres, but in polymyositis they may migrate to the centre. In treated disease, variations in muscle fibre diameter remain, but the infiltrate is reduced or absent. Later in the disease, muscle fibrosis may be extensive.

240 demonstrates a normal muscle biopsy, which is stained with haematoxylin and eosin. 241 shows an untreated case of polymyositis. Note the inflammatory cells lying between the muscle fibres, and the much greater variation in muscle fibre diameter. Central migration of the nuclei is apparent in some fibres. The patient shown in 242 had much more severe disease and the changes are correspondingly more gross. She responded well to high doses of corticosteroids and azathioprine.

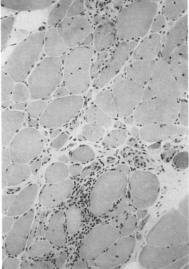

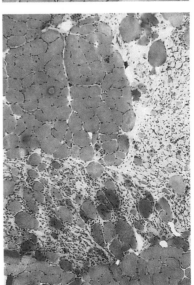

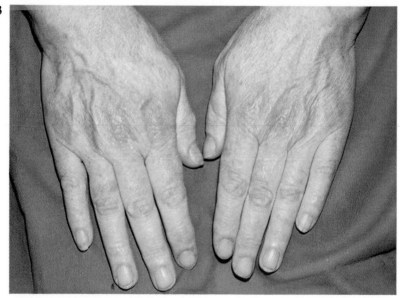

243 **243 Cutaneous changes in the hands in dermatomyositis.** Cutaneous changes are variable and not always present, but they are most typically seen in the hands. Purple-red, raised patches (due to vasculitis) affect the extensor surfaces of the finger joints and, occasionally, those of the elbows and knees. Later they may become atrophic. They are often called collodion patches. Nail fold capillary abnormalities (*see* **226**) and ragged cuticles are also seen. The siting of the erythema over the knuckles is typical of polymyositis/dermatomyositis and distinguishes it from SLE, in which a rash may develop over the proximal phalanges.

244   **245**

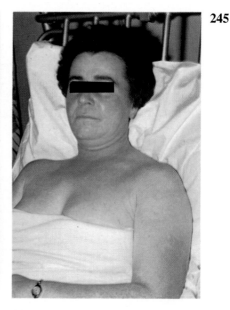

244 & 245 Facial rash of dermatomyositis. About 50% of patients develop a typical facial rash, with heliotrope (purple) discoloration and oedema of the eyelids. There may also be a 'butterfly' distribution across the bridge of the nose and upper cheeks, which reflects light exposure and may lead to confusion with SLE. Typical skin changes in the hands and significant muscle weakness are features of polymyositis/dermatomyositis but, if doubt exists, a muscle biopsy should be considered (*see* p.104) and is usually diagnostic.

246 Calcinosis in dermatomyositis. Calcinotic deposits around joints occur in younger patients with dermatomyositis. Here they are visible around the knee, and there is incipient ulceration of the skin. Severe vasculitic ulceration also arises in younger patients and scarring frequently results. Calcinotic deposits in muscle may occur, which are difficult to treat and potentially disabling.

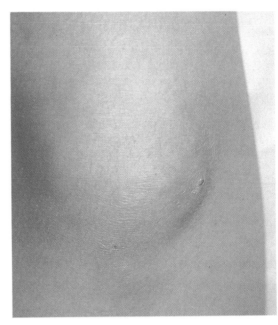

Management of polymyositis and dermatomyositis

Muscle disease should be monitored by regular formal strength testing and by serial measurements of the serum CPK levels. If the onset is acute, and in juvenile disease, initial hospitalisation is mandatory. Rest is important; the limbs should be supported by splinting. The use of corticosteroids has greatly improved the clinical outlook in childhood disease and in some adults. Those cases with an associated malignancy or with involvement of the respiratory or pharyngeal muscles have a worse prognosis.

The actual dose of corticosteroids to be used remains controversial. In children, after an initial daily dose of 1–2 mg/kg, dose reductions should be made on alternate days in order to prevent growth retardation. In adults an initial dose of at least 60 mg per day is usually needed for a few months. As strength improves and the tests return to normal, the dose can be gradually reduced. Maintenance of high doses can lead to corticosteroid-induced myopathy (and other Cushingoid changes) complicating the interpretation of muscle weakness. If a poor response to corticosteroids occurs, cytotoxic agents such as azathioprine should be added to the treatment regime. This is also important as an agent to maintain some patients on a lower dose of corticosteroids – a steroid sparing agent. Once the acute phase has settled, a graded regime of physiotherapy helps to restore strength and to avoid contracture formation. The disease sometimes persists for years and should be managed with the lowest maintenance doses of corticosteroids and/or cytotoxic agents possible.

Cutaneous involvement usually responds to corticosteroids, although antimalarials may suffice, particularly if the muscle disease is mild or controlled. Subcutaneous calcinotic deposits in juveniles may discharge and heal, resolve or require surgery. Deeper deposits in myofascial planes remain difficult to treat and potentially disabling.

Sjögren's syndrome

Sjögren's syndrome exists in a primary form, but it more commonly occurs in association with a wide variety of autoimmune disorders including RA, SLE, scleroderma, polymyositis and Graves' disease. Its clinical features are described in Chapter 2 (*see* **98–100**). In the primary disease, there is generally much more severe impairment of exocrine function. In some patients, massive swelling of the salivary glands arises, occasionally leading to the later development of a lymphoma. In its primary form it is associated with antibodies to the extractable nuclear antigen La, and with anti-Ro in the secondary form when complicating SLE.

Overlap syndromes and mixed connective tissue disease (MCTD)

Although there is a natural tendency to try to classify and subdivide diseases, this is not always possible. The term 'overlap syndrome' is used for the variety of patients who demonstrate features of two (occasionally three) of the autoimmune disorders. Almost every possible combination has been reported, but the most common are: a mixed picture of RA and SLE; RA or SLE with Sjögren's syndrome; and scleroderma or SLE with polymyositis. Other organ-specific autoimmune diseases, such as autoimmune thyroiditis or vitiligo, may also occur. Treatment is determined by the individual clinical picture.

The term 'mixed connective tissue disease' (MCTD) has been used to describe patients, usually female, who present with puffy swelling of the hands, Raynaud's phenomenon, polyarthritis, myositis and oesophageal dysfunction. It was thought to have a relatively good prognosis. Most unusually, the disease was initially defined on immunological grounds by the presence of autoantibodies (eventually found to be antibodies against ribonuclear protein) which produced speckled antinuclear staining (*see* **Table 13**). The specificity of these autoantibodies to define the syndrome is no longer accepted, however, and its prognosis is not always good. Indeed, many physicians doubt that MCTD is anything other than another overlap syndrome!

Polyarteritis nodosa and vasculitis

The clinical spectrum of vasculitic disease is wide. In many cases the vasculitis, which is an inflammation of the vascular walls, complicates another disease, for example, RA or the other connective tissue disorders described above. The disease falls into two broad groups: necrotising vasculitis and giant cell arteritis. In necrotising vasculitis the infiltration is mainly with polymorphonuclear leucocytes, and there is fibrinoid necrosis of vessel walls. Large or medium muscular arteries, small arteries, venules or arterioles may be predominantly affected, and different clinical syndromes result according to which vessel type is affected. In giant cell arteritis, there is a more focal pattern of inflammation, associated with granuloma formation. A specific type of vasculitis of large arteries occurs in temporal arteritis (giant cell arteritis) (*see* **302 & 303**). In most cases of systemic vasculitis, antibodies to cytoplasmic components of neutrophils (antineutrophil-cytoplasmic antibodies – *see* **Table 13**), detectable either as perinuclear or granular staining, can be demonstrated.

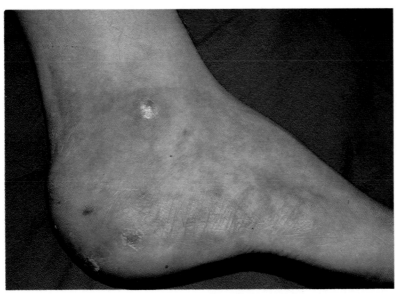

247 Polyarteritis nodosa (PAN) demonstrating livedo reticularis and ulceration. PAN, a vasculitis predominantly of large and medium muscular arteries, presents in individuals over 40 years of age, with nonspecific fever, malaise and weight loss. It may mimic a carcinomatous myopathy or polymyalgia rheumatica (*see* p.135), but the important clinical clues are myalgia, weakness due to mononeuritis multiplex, and patchy sensory abnormalities. Cutaneous involvement may occur, with painful, chronic ulceration and, occasionally, livedo reticularis in which the lattice-work patterning seen in the skin is due to a venulitis. Both conditions are seen here.

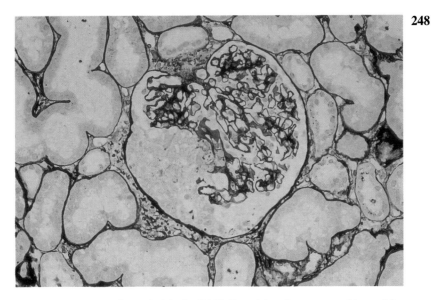

248

248 Focal glomerulonephritis in PAN. Renal involvement, evidenced by proteinuria or casts in a fresh specimen of urine, is common in PAN. Hypertension may result. This biopsy, from a patient with microscopic polyarteritis, is stained with hexamine silver and shows segmental necrotising glomerulonephritis with crescent formation. Unaffected parts of the glomerulus look surprisingly normal, a typical finding in PAN. The patient presented with fever and malaise, was hypertensive and had microscopic haematuria.

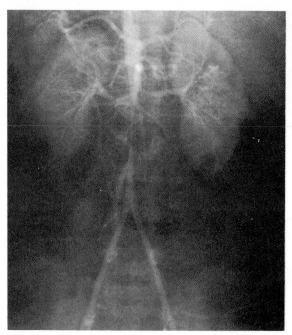

249 Takayasu's arteritis. Also known as pulseless disease, this disease is an inflammatory arteritis of the aorta and large and medium arteries. There is usually a generalised malaise, myalgia and fever. Typically, the pulses of the upper limbs are diminished or absent. Teenage girls and young women are affected. This aortogram (from a girl) shows marked tapering of the abdominal aorta due to aortitis. Femoral pulses were absent. The ESR is usually very raised and there may be a neutrophilia, but there are no specific blood tests. Angiography is diagnostic, and treatment is with high dose corticosteroids (with or without cytotoxic therapy). Early diagnosis and treatment usually leads to a good prognosis.

250

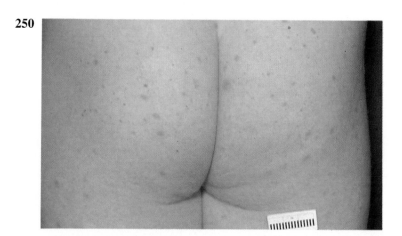

250 Henoch–Schoenlein purpura. Also known as anaphylactoid or allergic purpura, this condition generally presents in young boys who have had a recent upper respiratory tract infection. A characteristic maculopapular, purpuric rash generally develops over the buttocks and legs, as shown here. This boy also has subcutaneous oedema. Other clinical features may include arthralgia, arthritis, abdominal pain and gastrointestinal bleeding (rarely massive) and, occasionally, the nephrotic syndrome. There is a characteristic histologial picture of venulitis and IgA deposition in the lesions.

251 Wegener's granulomatosis. Although the spectrum of clinical features in Wegener's granulomatosis is very wide, involvement of the upper and lower respiratory tracts is the most common presenting problem. Sinusitis, nasal blockage or discharge, or shortness of breath (with pulmonary infiltrates on the chest X-ray) all occur. Patients may also develop arthritis or mild to fulminant glomerulonephritis. Diagnosis is usually made by direct biopsy of the granulomata in the nasopharynx or lungs. The finding of granulomata is necessary to confirm the diagnosis, but it can also be inferred, as in this patient, from the finding of erosion of the bony walls of the nasal sinuses and nasal septum (arrows). Granulomatous tissue in the right sinus appears white on this MRI scan and is more florid than would be seen with other causes of mucosal hypertrophy.

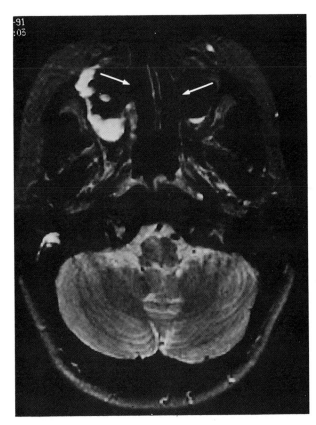

Management

Corticosteroids, often administered in combination with cytotoxic drugs such as azathioprine or cyclophosphamide, have transformed the outlook of many of the vasculitic disorders. Their use depends upon the severity of the disease and its type. Thus, in Henloch–Schoenlein purpura, only symptomatic treatment with NSAIDs is usually indicated, as the disease is self-limiting in most cases. Corticosteroids may be needed, however, if nephrotic syndrome develops.

In PAN, corticosteroids are generally required. They are frequently used in combination with a cytotoxic drug, which acts as a steroid-sparing agent, reducing the steroid dose and, thus, the risk of osteoporosis in these often elderly patients. In Wegener's granulomatosis, treatment with cyclophosphamide and steroids has radically improved the prognosis: this previously fatal disease is now curable in up to 90% of patients. If cyclophosphamide is to be used in the younger patient, advice about sperm-banking and fertility is obligatory. Specialist care is essential.

8 Arthritis in childhood

Juvenile chronic arthritis

The name of George Frederic Still has been eponymously linked with juvenile chronic arthritis (JCA) since his initial description of cases in 1897. However, the label 'Still's disease' is now best restricted to a particular variant, which is better called systemic-onset juvenile chronic arthritis. Several different classifications of JCA have been proposed, but it is generally agreed that to qualify, symptoms should start before 16 years of age and the disease should last for more than 3 months. Most classifications are essentially clinical, although serological tests and HLA type are important adjuncts.

A more extensive discussion is beyond the scope of this Atlas; the aim here is to remind the practitioner of the importance of recognising the possibility of arthritis in a child and of referring cases early to a specialist paediatric rheumatologist. Patients and their families frequently need a great deal of support, not only from the medical profession, but also from specialist physiotherapists, occupational therapists, teachers and, occasionally, from specialist orthopaedic surgeons. This support is best provided, whenever possible, by a team working in a unit dedicated to childhood arthritis.

Juvenile arthritis is rare. Boys and girls are equally affected by the systemic disease between 1 and 5 years of age, after which there is a female preponderance. A pauciarticular pattern of arthritis affects girls between the ages of 1 and 9 years, and they are at risk of developing chronic iridocyclitis. Pauciarticular disease in older children is usually of the seronegative or spondylitic type. It may be associated, usually at a later stage, with the development of psoriasis, inflammatory bowel disease, or typical sacroiliitis and spondylitis: these children may be HLA B27-positive.

In young children a limp or failure to move a limb, even in the absence of obvious distress due to pain, may indicate arthritis or other joint or bony problems (such as an infective arthritis of the hip, or a malignancy), and should not be ignored.

Systemic-onset juvenile chronic arthritis (Still's disease)

Table 14. Major clinical features of systemic juvenile arthritis

High, swinging pyrexia

Evanescent, pink macular rash

Arthralgia and myalgia

Generalised lymphadenopathy

Splenomegaly and hepatomegaly

Pericarditis

Pleurisy (rare)

Episodic pauciarticular or chronic polyarticular arthritis develops eventually in some affected children

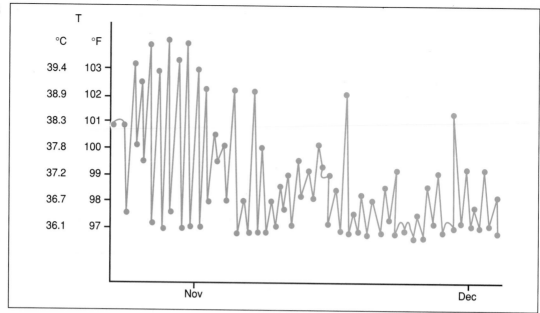

252

Nov   Dec

252 Temperature chart of early systemic juvenile arthritis. Fever is the usual presenting feature of systemic juvenile arthritis. It is remittent and dramatic, often peaking (at up to 40°C) in the early evening and settling over night. During the febrile episode, the child is very unwell, with an obvious rash, but as the fever subsides, the rash fades and well-being improves remarkably. There is a typical, although nonspecific, response to aspirin or an NSAID such as naproxen (ibuprofen in the under fives). The pyrexia differs from that of rheumatic fever, which demonstrates less dramatic swings and is usually sustained.

253

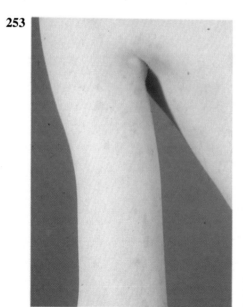

254

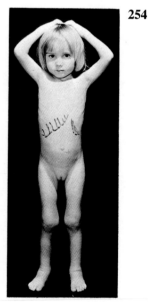

253 Rash of systemic juvenile arthritis. Seen mainly in the evening as the fever flares, or after a hot bath, the rash comprises small, generally nonitchy, red macules, which sometimes have a paler centre. The macules disappear and reappear, but do not spread to form the typical marginate erythema of rheumatic fever (*see* **269**).

254 Hepatosplenomegaly in systemic disease. Lymphadenopathy is a common feature of the active phase of the disease and is usually proximal to inflamed joints. It may be gross and visible. Histology is nonspecific, but biopsy may be necessary to distinguish the disease from leukaemia or malignancy. Hepatosplenomegaly is found in the more severely affected child.

255 Arthritis in systemic disease. In the early stages of the systemic-onset disease, arthralgia is frequent. Arthritis is usually mild, occurring later in the disease in 50% of cases. The cervical spine is typically affected and restriction of neck movement is an important clinical sign. There is a tendency for this neck involvement to progress to upper cervical fusion, initially of the apophyseal joints, eventually involving the vertebral bodies (as shown here). Peripheral joint arthritis develops later as an acute polyarthritis, which may become chronic, or as an episodic pauciarticular arthritis, predominantly affecting hips and knees (*see* p.118).

(**Adult-onset Still's disease**, with fever, lymphadenopathy, hepatosplenomegaly and arthritis is rare, but the diagnosis should be considered, particularly if the clinical picture is consistent and serological tests are negative. It is difficult to treat and has a generally poor prognosis).

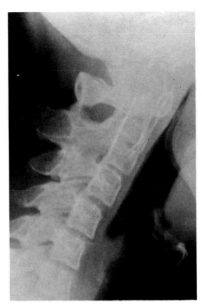

Polyarticular-onset juvenile chronic arthritis

A polyarticular pattern of presentation can occur at any age, from the first year onwards. It is more common in girls than in boys. In a proportion of cases, it is preceded by the systemic disease described in the previous section.

Serological tests for rheumatoid factor are almost invariably negative. In a teenage girl, polyarticular arthritis and a strongly positive rheumatoid factor indicate that she has juvenile onset RA.

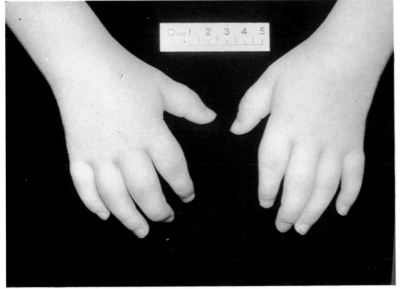

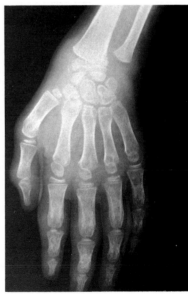

256 & 257 Acute polyarticular arthritis in systemic juvenile arthritis. There is usually symmetrical involvement of the hands and wrists, with the PIP joints predominantly affected in the fingers. There is often marked flexor tenosynovitis. The DIP joints are sometimes involved, distinguishing this disease from juvenile RA. Joint swelling is often gross, but is frequently associated with a disproportionate lack of pain and tenderness.

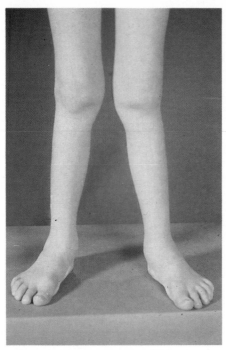

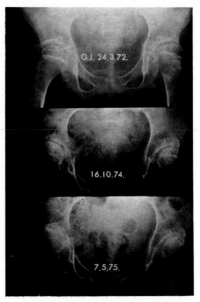

259 Progressive arthritis of the hips. The degree of joint destruction that may occur in this disease is demonstrated in these serial X-rays taken over a 3-year period. The hips of a child with persistently active disease are illustrated. Eventual total hip replacement at a young age is inevitable; it will restore mobility as long as other lower limb joints are not destroyed.

258 Polyarticular arthritis. Early involvement of the knees and ankles also occurs, and the cervical spine, temporomandibular joints and hips are sometimes affected. Progression to severe joint damage is more common in the adolescent.

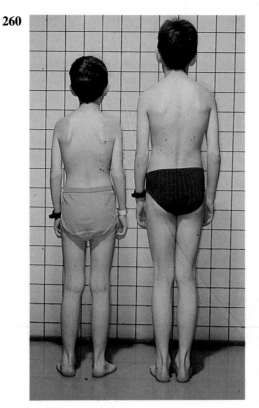

260 Generalised growth retardation in JCA. A variety of growth disturbances can occur in polyarticular-onset JCA. General stunting of growth may be due to the severity and chronicity of the disease, and/or the need to use corticosteroids in the more severe cases. Steroid-induced growth retardation can be prevented or reduced if alternative daily doses can be administered effectively. In this case the twin on the left had systemic-onset disease, followed by 5 years of polyarthritis which required a period on corticosteroids, although he was not taking them at the time of the picture.

261 Underdevelopment of the jaw (micrognathia). Premature fusion of the epiphyses of the mandible is due to associated temporomandibular joint disease. Fusion of the joint itself is unusual, but the resultant underdevelopment of the lower jaw leads to severe bite problems and this typical facial appearance.

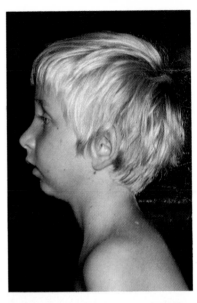

262 Metaphyseal overgrowth in juvenile polyarthritis. When the knee is involved in polyarticular disease, there is often overgrowth of the femoral epiphyses and widening of the intercondylar notch.

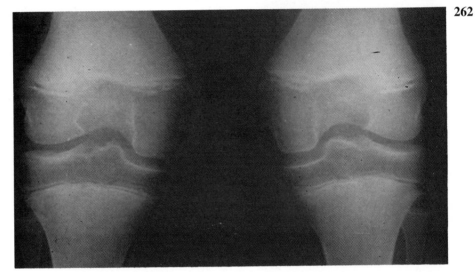

263 Premature fusion of the epiphyseal plate. Early fusion of the epiphysis may lead to shortening of a leg or of the fingers or toes. Here, there has been rapid fusion of the epiphysis at the proximal end of the proximal phalanx of the affected right great toe, over an 8-month period.

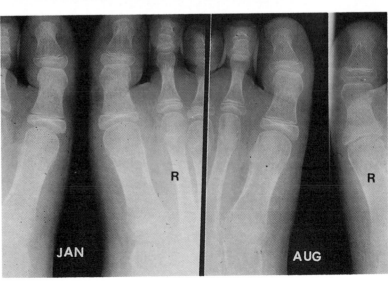

Pauciarticular-onset juvenile chronic arthritis

The most common mode of onset of JCA is pauci-articular and causes the least systemic upset. It is defined as affecting 4 or fewer joints within the first 6 months of onset. The larger joints, especially of the lower limb, are affected, often asymmetrically. Occasionally, there is slow progression to an asymmetrical polyarthritis. Teenage boys who present with lower limb arthritis, frequently have a family history of psoriasis, AS or other seronegative arthritides (*see* Chapter 6) and show an increased frequency of HLA B27. They may later develop these conditions themselves, and are at risk of developing acute anterior uveitis (*see* **191**).

Preteenage girls with pauciarticular JCA form a separate group, which is at high risk of developing chronic eye involvement. Younger children with a pauciarticular onset of disease should always be tested for antinuclear antibodies. A positive test indicates an increased risk, but they must be referred to an oph-thalmologist for a 3–4-monthly slit-lamp examination, even if the antibody is negative, because of the risk of insidious development of chronic iridocyclitis (*see* **266 & 267**).

x

264
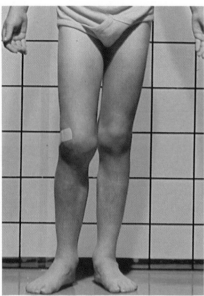
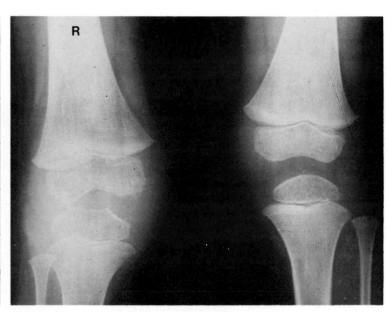
26

264 & 265 Asymmetrical arthritis in a teenage boy. Older boys most commonly present with a monarthritis of the knee. This may be a manifestation of juvenile spondylitis or psoriatic arthritis. Often, the spondylitis does not develop until the early twenties; only then will the sacroiliac joints and spine become radiologically abnormal. This 11-year-old boy had arthritis of the knee and ankle predominantly, with minimal inflammation of the left elbow. Involvement of the knee may lead to overgrowth both of the metaphysis and the epiphysis, here seen in his right knee (**265**). Deformity can result, which may require later osteotomy.

266
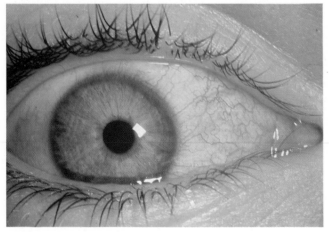

266 Early chronic iridocyclitis. Younger, preteenage children, particularly girls, may present with pauciarticular arthritis. They are usually positive for antinuclear antibodies and are at risk of developing chronic anterior iridocyclitis. Because there is often little obvious inflammation of the eye, unless it is carefully looked for, and pain may not be significant (in marked contrast to the severe pain and obvious redness seen in acute anterior iritis), the problem can be easily overlooked until it is too late. Early and regular slit-lamp examinations are essential in all preteenage children with pauciarticular disease. Punctate precipitates on the posterior surface of the cornea are the earliest feature. Eye involvement frequently becomes bilateral, but this usually happens within a year of the first eye being affected, rarely later.

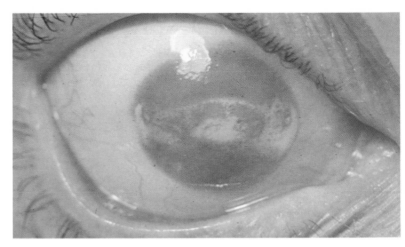

267 Band keratopathy and cataract due to chronic iridocyclitis. Chronic iridocyclitis requires early specialist treatment, but is often difficult to control. Band keratopathy (a band of opacity across the cornea) and a cataract may develop, leading to blindness. Glaucoma may also occur.

Juvenile onset seropositive rheumatoid arthritis

A few older girls present with polyarthritis in their early to mid teens and are found to have a positive rheumatoid factor. The disease is treated as a juvenile onset of RA. It may lead to severe joint damage, although a proportion of cases eventually goes into remission.

Management of juvenile chronic arthritis

Referral to a specialist centre is mandatory. The importance of teamwork and counselling has already been stressed. Splinting and rest, with appropriate exercise once the inflammation settles, are all essential for the best possible prognosis. Despite sometimes prolonged hospitalisation, it is important to maintain a child's education. In the longer term, especially if the disease persists despite drug treatment, the advice of an expert paediatric orthopaedic surgeon may be needed. Rehabilitation programmes and specific aids can do much to improve the quality of life of even the most severely disabled children giving them the chance of a more normal adult life.

Drug treatment is the mainstay of management of both the acute and the progressive disease. In the initial stages, pain and fever can be alleviated with relatively high doses of soluble aspirin (up to 70 mg/kg/day), but the risk of liver damage due to Reye's syndrome makes it preferable to use either paracetamol or appropriate doses of an NSAID such as naproxen (ibuprofen in the under fives). Corticosteroids are used sparingly, but may be needed in children with severe systemic JCA or progressive inflammatory joint disease which is not helped by NSAIDs, and in cases of chronic iridocyclitis. In the latter, topical steroids should be tried first. If systemic steroids are used, the dose should be reduced on an alternate-day basis as soon as possible to prevent growth retardation and other side-effects. Local corticosteroid injections are useful in pauciarticular disease, but they may have to be given under a light general anaesthetic.

The use of second-line drugs is sometimes necessary. Because of the significant risk of inducing leukaemia, cytotoxic agents are used only in the presence of amyloidosis in the more severely affected child.

Rheumatic fever and poststreptococcal arthritis

Rheumatic fever is an important childhood disease in the developing countries of Africa, Asia and South America, but rare in Europe, North America and Australasia, having declined since the 1920s, after a peak incidence at the turn of the century. The decline predated the development of antibiotics and may have been due to improvements in hygiene and social conditions, or to a decrease in the virulence of the causative organism. Rheumatic fever has an important long-term morbidity and mortality due to cardiac involvement. Recent reports suggest that it may be reappearing in developed countries.

Generally, children are affected for the first time between the ages of 4 and 15 years, with a peak incidence at 7–8 years. First time occurences in adults are rare.

Rheumatic fever, which may involve the joints, skin, heart and brain, is preceded by a sore throat due to a group A ß-haemolytic Streptococcus; in recent years, throat cultures have rarely proved positive, however, because of the delay in onset of the symptoms, and the prior use of antibiotics in most patients. Occasionally, the infection arises elsewhere, from, for example, an infected skin ulcer. A rising titre of antistreptolysin-O antibodies is suggestive. Once individuals have been affected, each further infection by the same organism carries the risk of a recurrence.

The delayed manifestations of the disease develop 1–5 weeks after the initial infection. They are due to antibodies which cross-react with human sarcolemma and with cardiac or brain tissue. A variety of factors appears to contribute to susceptibility. There is an interesting negative association with blood group O, and a positive association with nonsecretors of the ABO blood groups.

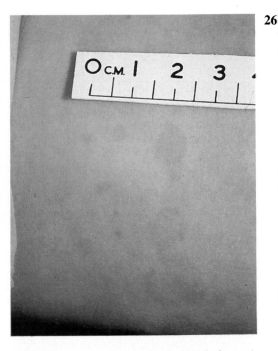

268 Arthritis in rheumatic fever. Fever is persistent and less high than that seen in systemic juvenile chronic arthritis (*see* **252**). Also in contrast with systemic-onset disease, the arthritis starts at the same time as the fever. Joint pain, swelling and redness, usually of the larger joints, are marked, and the arthritis characteristically migrates from joint to joint, each being affected for a few days if untreated. This child has an inflamed knee and a typical rash.

269 Erythema marginatum in rheumatic fever. A small proportion of cases demonstrate the typical spreading rash of erythema marginatum, which, as shown here, has a red, serpiginous border and central pallor. Crops of small subcutaneous nodules may occur over the bony prominences and the tendons.

Carditis and Sydenham's chorea in rheumatic fever

Pericarditis and/or acute myocarditis may complicate rheumatic fever and cause heart failure. A marked tachycardia suggests myocarditis. Careful cardiac examination and an ECG are essential. A prolonged PR interval and other rhythm disturbances may occur. With time, and especially after recurrent attacks, the heart valves (particularly the mitral and aortic) become stenotic. This occurs in up to 50% of individuals who develop carditis, and is the cause of significant long-term morbidity. Recurrent attacks lead to a worse prognosis. Unrecognised rheumatic heart disease may lead to high-output congestive failure during pregnancy. Prior to the use of antibiotics, death was commonly due to subacute bacterial endocarditis, but severe valvular disease can now be managed surgically.

Sydenham's chorea develops in girls after a greater delay than the carditis, with which it may coexist. It is characterised by purposeless, uncoordinated movements, restlessness and inattention. The movements tend to settle during sleep. Chorea may last for several months and relapses may occur over several years, but it appears to have no long-term sequelae.

Management of rheumatic fever

Bedrest is essential for the acutely ill child. Fever and arthritis can be controlled readily with salicylates, although care should be exercised owing to the risk of producing Reye's syndrome, and NSAIDs are preferable. Corticosteroids are increasingly being used in the carditis of rheumatic fever, because it is self-limiting and thus does not require prolonged treatment, with the resultant side-effects. Once the acute episode has settled, patients will require prophylactic penicillin throughout their childhood and teenage years.

9 Miscellaneous arthropathies and other nonarticular rheumatic disorders

In addition to those rheumatic disorders described in the preceeding chapters, which frequently present with pain and stiffness or frank arthritis as the primary complaints, there is a wide variety of other conditions which may cause rheumatic symptoms. The clinician must be constantly on the lookout for atypical patterns of pain or other symtoms which may indicate that a more unusual cause or an additional diagnosis should be sought. The list is large. This chapter describes a variety of diseases or situations in which joint involvement or musculo-skeletal symptoms are not uncommon, and which may first present to a rheumatologist or as a rheumatological complaint.

Traumatic lesions of the knee

270

271

272

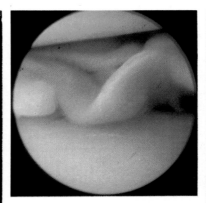

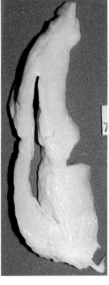

270–272 Torn medial meniscus. The most common cause of joint pain is trauma. If the synovial membrane is damaged or a meniscus of the knee torn, the result is acute pain and swelling. Intra-articular trauma may lead to haemarthrosis, but within a few days or weeks the effusion changes to a clear yellow. Rest, analgesia and aspiration help in the acute phase, followed by exercises to restore muscle power. Recurrence, or the presence of episodes of locking of the knee joint, warrants further investigation and, if available, MRI is a noninvasive investigation which can clearly demonstrate meniscal tears. Here (**270**), there is a large tear of the posterior horn of the medial meniscus, extending to its lower surface (arrow). The signal from the lateral meniscus is normal.

Although it is invasive, arthroscopy by an experienced surgeon is often the investigation of choice, offering the chance not only to visualise the lesion, but also to remove a damaged meniscus or a loose body, or to biopsy any abnormal synovium. The arthroscopic appearance of a longitudinal tear in the medial meniscus (a bucket handle tear) is shown in **271**, with the operative specimen illustrated in **272**.

273

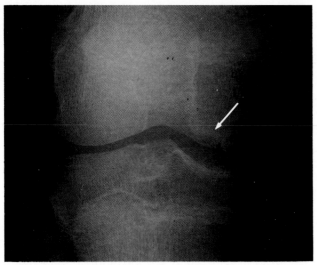

273 Osteochondritis dissecans (transchondral fracture). Transchondral fracture most frequently occurs in adolescence; it may cause no symptoms, or pain, clicking and/or locking. An effusion may also develop. Trauma and genetic factors appear to be important in the aetiology. The most common site in an adolescent is the inner aspect of the medial femoral condyle (arrow), as seen in this 16-year-old with intermittent knee pain and swelling. Treatment is conservative, and revascularisation often occurs. If the fragment separates and causes locking, it should be removed. Other sites affected include the lateral femoral condyle (more commonly in older individuals), the patella and the talus.

Haemophilia

Haemophiliac patients who do not have access to factor VIII may suffer recurrent bleeds into their joints and the surrounding soft tissues, with or without trauma as a precipitating cause. Recurrent haemarthroses lead to severe destruction of the joint, and intramuscular bleeding produces secondary fibrous contractures.

Knees, ankles, elbows and shoulders are the most commonly affected joints. Prompt treatment with factor VIII, analgesia, aspiration of the joint and rest is vital. Physiotherapy is essential to prevent contractures and to maintain muscle strength once the acute episode has settled.

274

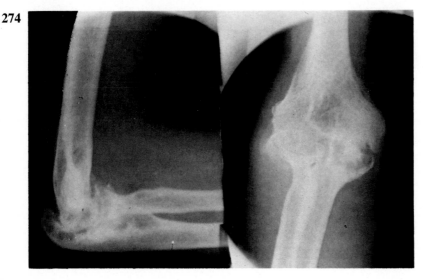

274 The elbow of a patient with haemophilia. The elbow joint is severely disrupted, with loss of joint space, patchy sclerosis, osteophytosis and cyst formation.

Haemoglobinopathies

The most common of the haemoglobinopathies is sickle-cell disease. It can cause a variety of joint and bone problems:

- Arthralgia and/or synovitis may occur during an acute sickle crisis.

- Aseptic necrosis of bone (*see* **312–314**) can develop, due to thrombosis of nutrient vessels.
- Osteomyelitis or septic arthritis may occur, usually due to Salmonella spp.

Pigmented villonodular synovitis

275 Haemarthrosis in pigmented villonodular synovitis. This monarthritis of unknown cause usually presents with an insidious onset of pain and swelling. The symptoms persist. Acute exacerbations are caused by intra-articular bleeding, when the aspirate is frankly bloody as here, or dark brown due to haemosiderin. The primary lesion is an area of synovium which is thrown up into multiple villi. It becomes pigmented brown due to haemosiderin deposition. Untreated, local damage to cartilage and bone occurs, eventually becoming radiologically apparent. Complete excision and/or radiotherapy are necessary to prevent damage and recurrence. Secondary osteoarthritis may supervene.

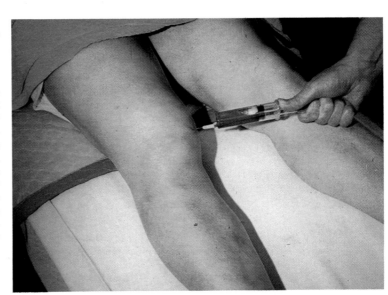

275

Gonococcal arthritis

Most gonococcal infections are treated early and complications are uncommon. Ineffective control of the infection may be related to the fact that it is occasionally asymptomatic, usually in women, or that individuals may default from treatment or acquire antibiotic-resistant strains of the organism. If gonococcaemia develops, the patient becomes febrile and develops arthralgias. Characteristic pustules, which may haemorrhage or ulcerate, develop on the distal extremities. Asymmetrical tenosynovitis and synovitis of wrists, fingers, knees or ankles can also occur. Even if it is untreated, the gonococcaemia may resolve, but some patients go on to develop a painful infective monarthritis. Occasionally, acute gonococcal arthritis develops without this prodromal septicaemic illness.

Organisms (gram-negative intracellular diplococci) can be cultured from the pustules early in the disease, and from septic joints. If gonorrhoea is suspected, infected joint fluid is best cultured in standard blood-culture bottles. Antibiotic sensitivities must be determined. Patients with disseminated disease should be admitted to hospital. Appropriate intravenous antibiotics are given until improvement is seen, followed by 1–3 weeks of oral treatment.

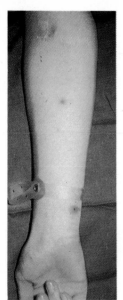

276 Gonococcal septicaemic skin lesions. These typical lesions appear on the distal limbs during early gonococcaemia. Between 3 and 20 such lesions are usual. The advice of a specialist in genitourinary medicine should be sought. Other genitourinary diseases may also be present, and appropriate examinations should be undertaken. This patient also has a flexor tenosynovitis of the fingers.

277 Gonococcal arthritis of the knee. This female patient developed an acute febrile illness and pustules which she ignored. Seven days later she was severely ill, with an acutely painful knee. The joint was hot and red, and aspiration produced copious amounts of pus containing gonococci. Early treatment with high doses of suitable antibiotics (in this case penicillin G 10 million units IV daily for 5 days, and then ampicillin 500 mg four times daily for 2 weeks) prevented potential long-term joint destruction.

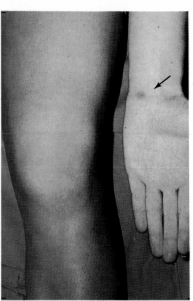

Acquired immunodeficiency syndrome (AIDS)

The recent epidemic of HIV infection, with AIDS developing in many, if not all, infected individuals, has brought with it many new clinical problems. Although not a major feature, arthritis may be the first manifestation of the disease: an acute mono- or pauciarticular inflammatory arthritis occurs, sometimes with an acute onset of cutaneous psoriasis (or a flare of pre-existing psoriasis). Interestingly, the profound depletion of T-helper lymphocytes does not reduce the inflammatory aspects of the arthritis. Sacroiliitis also arises in some individuals, who may go on to develop ankylosing spondylitis. In addition, there is an apparently increased incidence of pain arising at tendon insertions (for example, tennis elbow), and/or other problems such as trochanteric bursitis. The pain of these rheumatological manifestations may be particularly difficult to control, even with high doses of NSAIDs.

Of the malignancies that appear to be associated with AIDS, lymphoma is one of the more common, and may present with bone pain or cause focal neurological deficits.

The most serious rheumatic complication of HIV and AIDS is an infective arthritis, which may be more insidious in onset in these immunosuppressed patients than in others. Any inflamed joint in an individual who is HIV-positive or has established AIDS should be aspirated early, under careful sterile conditions to protect both the patient and the doctor. The advice of a bacteriologist should always be sought immediately, in order to ensure that the cultures include media and conditions suitable for the detection of atypical organisms, as well as the more common ones.

The early and effective treatment of opportunistic infections in AIDS contributes greatly to the prolongation of life, and all medical practitioners must now include infection in their differential diagnosis of new problems presenting in known AIDS cases or in at-risk individuals. Possible HIV infection should never be forgotten, particularly when the arthritis is atypical, the pain severe, or the patient is generally unwell or has skin problems and is in a high-risk group.

278 & 279 Infective arthritis in a patient known to be HIV-positive. This HIV-positive patient, who had a small area of Kaposi's sarcoma on one leg, presented with an acutely painful foot and a small pustule overlying the metatarsal region. The X-ray (**278**) shows destruction of the second MTP joint, and the scan (**279**) confirms increased radio-isotope uptake at this site. *Pseudomonas aeruginosa* was cultured from the pus. This acute episode reflected an underlying *Pseudomonas* septicaemia and, despite broad-spectrum antibiotic treatment, the patient died within a few days. Atypical organisms (including mycobacteria) may be found in such patients, and the bacteriologist should be alerted to these possibilities.

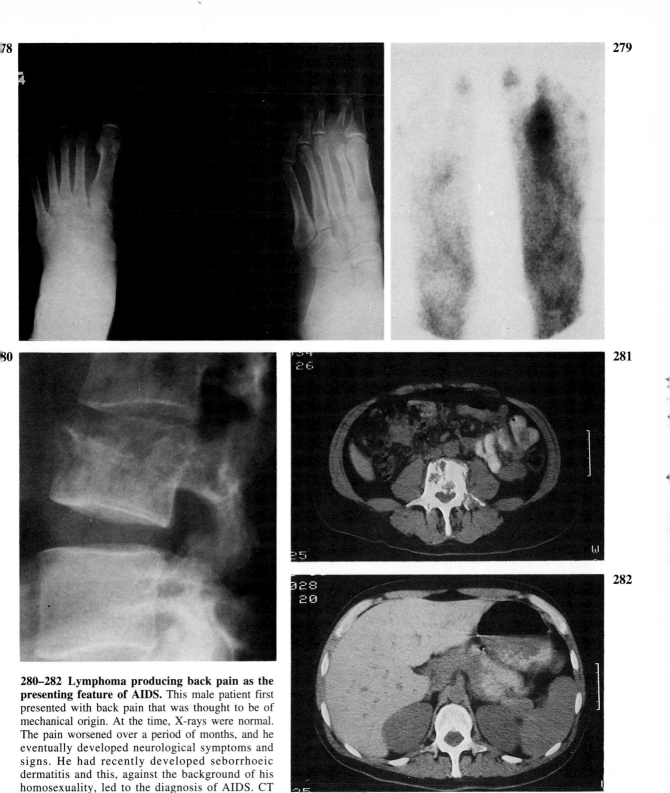

280–282 Lymphoma producing back pain as the presenting feature of AIDS. This male patient first presented with back pain that was thought to be of mechanical origin. At the time, X-rays were normal. The pain worsened over a period of months, and he eventually developed neurological symptoms and signs. He had recently developed seborrhoeic dermatitis and this, against the background of his homosexuality, led to the diagnosis of AIDS. CT scanning (**281**) revealed patchy destruction of the body and posterior elements of the third lumbar vertebra, and a needle biopsy confirmed the diagnosis of a lymphoma. He responded well to radiotherapy and chemotherapy, returning to work for 18 months, before he eventually died of other manifestations of AIDS. A normal CT scan of a lumbar vertebra (**282**) is included for comparison.

Lyme disease

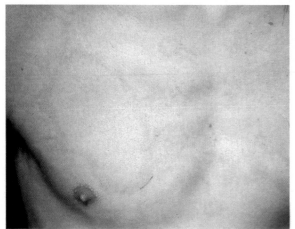

283 Erythema chronicum migrans. Although well described in the nineteenth century European medical literature, the recognition of Lyme disease during an epidemic in New England, together with the discovery of the causative organism, is a recent classic of medical detective work. The first sign of the disease is an expanding erythematous annular lesion of the skin, which lasts a few weeks. The patient is often febrile and complains of a headache. Occasionally, severe neurological or cardiac complications occur. About 25% of cases develop an acute pauciarticular arthritis, which resolves but may relapse. The disease is due to a spirochaete, *Borrelia burgdorferi*, and usually develops following a bite from an infected tick (*Ixodes* spp.). It can be diagnosed by the detection of specific antibodies, and responds well to penicillin or tetracycline.

The diabetic hand

Diabetic patients may develop a variety of hand problems, frequently in combination. These include:
- Nodular flexor tenosynovitis.
- Carpal tunnel syndrome (*see* **106 & 107**).
- Dupuytren's contracture.
- Diabetic sclerodactyly.
- Diabetic peripheral neuropathy.

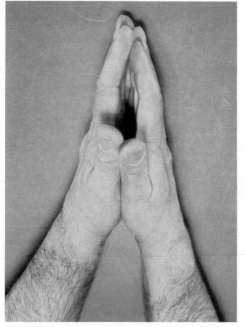

284 The 'prayer' sign. The diabetic stiff hand, which results in difficulty in apposing some or all of the fingers (a positive 'prayer' sign), requires careful examination. Probably the most common cause is coincidental mild nodal osteoarthritis. In the younger patient, nodular flexor tenosynovitis is more common, and may play a part in the generally asymptomatic inability to extend the fingers fully. It also produces morning stiffness of the fingers and 'trigger finger'. A Dupuytren's contracture may also contribute to a positive prayer sign. Trigger fingers and painful nodular tenosynovitis should be treated by injection of corticosteroids or, if persistent or troublesome, by surgery.

285 Diabetic sclerodactyly. In a small proportion of patients, thickening of the skin also occurs. As a result, it is difficult to pinch up a fold of skin on the back of the fingers. The skin becomes tight and shiny, and the appearance resembles that seen in scleroderma (*see* p.97). This finding is probably a reflection of poor diabetic control and is associated with an increased risk of vascular complications of diabetes.

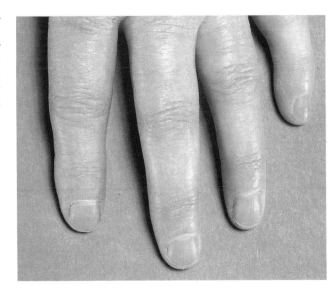

Acromegaly

Joint pain and muscle weakness are common features of acromegaly. Increased thickness of cartilage leads to widening of the joint spaces, visible on X-ray. There is a predisposition to early secondary osteoarthritis (*see* **139**), which is independent of adequate control of raised growth hormone levels, whether achieved by surgical or other means.

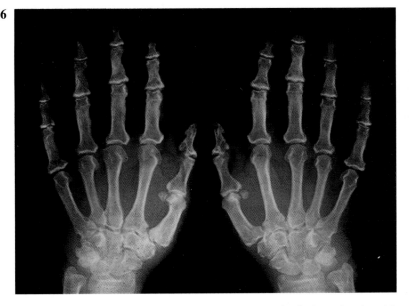

286 Acromegalic hands. This X-ray demonstrates typically large hands, with thickened soft tissues. Hypertrophic cartilage has increased the joint spaces, and there is prominent tufting of the terminal phalanges. Marginal osteophytes develop, together with ossification at muscle attachments.

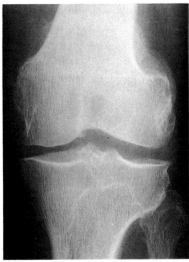

287 Acromegalic knee. As the patient is standing, the joint space on the X-ray accurately represents the thickness of the hypertrophic cartilage. (Caution: on a film of a knee joint that is not bearing weight, a large effusion may occasionally lead to apparent widening of the joint space in nonacromegalic patients.)

Myxoedema and Grave's disease

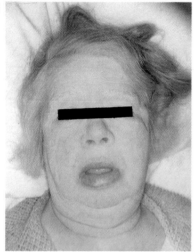

288 Myxoedema. A gradual onset of symptoms is typical of hypothyroidism. Before developing the more typical features of myxoedema, such as weight gain, cold intolerance, constipation or a change in facial appearance, patients may present with widespread nonspecific aches and pains. In such atypical cases the diagnosis is aided by maintaining a high index of suspicion, noting any previous history of thyroid disease, and looking for a low level of thyroxine and a raised level of thyroid stimulating' hormone (TSH) in the serum. There is a good response to thyroxine replacement.

Grave's disease

A rare complication, seen in patients with previous or current Grave's disease (autoimmune thyroiditis associated with autoantibodies to the TSH receptor or a closely related protein), is the development of painless thickening of the fingers, clubbing, exophthalmos and radiological evidence of 'fluffy' periostitis (thyroid acropachy). Bilateral firm dermal plaques over the tibiae (pretibial myxoedema) may also occur. These changes, which are due to local deposition of mucopolysaccharides, are self-limiting and not usually affected by correction of the thyroid status.

Hyperparathyroidism

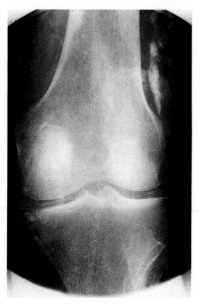

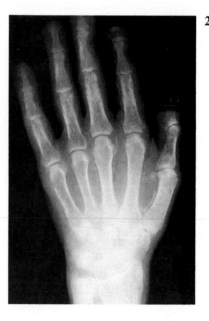

289 Chondrocalcinosis and soft-tissue calcification. Excess production of parathormone usually arises from an autonomous parathyroid adenoma (rarely a carcinoma). Secondary hyperparathyroidism is seen in chronic renal failure. It may be associated with joint pain due to acute pseudogout, which is secondary to chondrocalcinosis (*see* p.64). In this patient the obvious calcification of the menisci is associated with extensive soft-tissue calcification, a feature which distinguishes it from primary chondrocalcinosis.

290 Osteitis fibrosa cystica. The classic bone changes seen in long-standing hyperparathyroidism are illustrated, with resorption of the phalangeal tufts (best seen in index finger) and loss of definition of the bone margins due to subperiosteal resorption.

Osteoporosis

There are a number of risk factors for osteoporosis (*see* **Table 15**). In younger, asymptomatic women with several such factors, it is probably worth using hormone-replacement therapy and oral calcium supplements during the first 5–10 years after the menopause. Exercise and stopping smoking should be encouraged. Long-term studies, however, have not yet determined whether this approach will prevent, or even decrease, the risk of subsequent fracture, and the approach may itself have a significant morbidity. The use of 3-month cycles of doses of a diphosphonate for two weeks, followed by calcium supplementation for the rest of the 3-month period, may be helpful in preventing further osteoporotic fractures in symptomatic patients. The acute pain is reduced in some cases by a short course of calcitonin or of intravenous pamidronate.

Table 15. Risk factors for osteoporosis.

Female sex
Family history
Poor nutrition in teens and twenties
Inadequate exercise
Fair hair
Smoking
Early menopause
Slim habitus
Long-term corticosteroid treatment

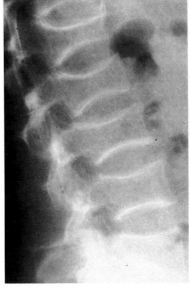

291

291 Postmenopausal osteoporosis. In osteoporosis, there is reduced bone mass, but normal mineralisation. Although the condition is itself asymptomatic, the patient is at increased risk of wrist, hip and spinal fractures after trauma, which may be minimal (*see* **164–166**). Any symptoms that do arise are due to such fractures and are seen in elderly women who have developed osteoporosis over a number of years. This patient's X-ray demonstrates reduced density of trabecular bone, thinning of the cortices, and typical biconcave vertebrae. There is a collapse fracture of the first lumbar vertebra (L1), but the pedicles are intact on the AP film (not shown), making an underlying malignancy less likely (compare **167 & 168**). If there is diagnostic doubt, clinical examination for a possible source of a secondary deposit is necessary and a bone scan may show multiple deposits. Biopsy of the affected bone may be required to clarify the diagnosis.

Osteomalacia and rickets

Osteomalacia is a disorder of bone mineralisation; the bone mass is usually normal. The primary abnormality is one of vitamin D deficiency and/or an irregularity in its metabolism to vitamin D3 in the kidney or in sunlight-exposed skin. The most common symptom is of diffuse skeletal aching. The patient may also complain of muscular weakness, mainly of proximal muscles, and have a waddling gait.

Table 16. Causes of osteomalacia.

Dietary deficiency
Malabsorption
Lack of exposure to sunlight
Renal failure
Phosphate-losing nephropathy
Long-term phenytoin treatment

292

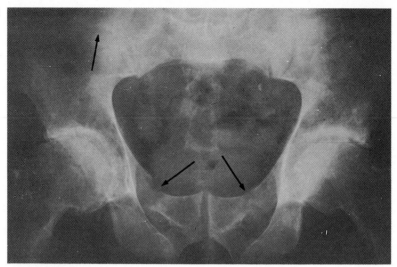

292 Looser's (transformation) zones in osteomalacia. Pathological pseudofractures and spinal vertebral collapse may lead to acute, localised pain. Typical sites of pseudofracture include the medial border of the femur and femoral neck, the pelvic rami, and the medial borders of the scapulae. These areas of linear demineralisation, which run at right angles to the cortex, are diagnostic. They are not always symptomatic. An X-ray of the pelvis is obligatory in suspected osteomalacia. This patient (who also has coincidental severe OA of the hips) demonstrates Looser's zones in both anterior pubic rami and in both iliac bones (arrows).

The diagnosis is also suggested by a moderately or greatly raised serum alkaline phosphatase (SAP) of bony origin. In severe cases, there may be hypocalcaemia, leading to tetany and a positive Trousseau's sign. Treatment is by dietary supplementation with vitamin D, or with vitamin D3 if renal disease is the cause.

293

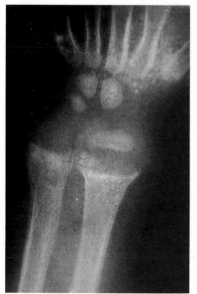

293 & 294 Childhood rickets. Childhood vitamin D deficiency leads to a different clinical picture, with bone tenderness and, if the diagnosis is delayed, deformity of the legs, arms, ribcage and skull. Muscle weakness is often prominent. In the growing skeleton, defective mineralisation occurs not only in bone but also in the cartilaginous matrix at the growth plate. On X-ray, there is obvious expansion and irregularity of the growth plates, visible here in the distal radius and ulna and in the proximal and distal tibia and fibula.

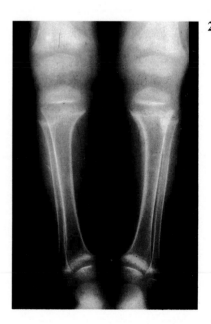

Paget's disease of bone (osteitis deformans)

The aetiology of Paget's disease is unknown, although viral inclusion bodies have been described. It shows a patchy geographical distribution, being relatively common in parts of the UK, but rare in Scandinavia. The incidence increases with advancing age. There is abnormal bone turnover and remodelling. Bone is excessively resorbed, and replaced with coarse, dense trabecular bone in a haphazard pattern. This leads to the typical radiological appearance of enlarged bones with patchy sclerosis and thickened cortices. There may be adjacent areas of lucency. Bone enlargement on X-ray is important in distinguishing Paget's disease from sclerotic secondary deposits from, for example, carcinoma of the breast or prostate.

Paget's disease is common in older people and gen-erally asymptomatic, often being found on X-rays that have been performed for other reasons. The serum alkaline phosphatase (SAP) is raised, as is the urinary hydroxyproline. Serum calcium, phosphate and acid phosphatase are all normal. Treatment depends upon the symptoms, which include those due to compression by the expanded bones, local bone pain and, occasionally, urinary calculi or high-output cardiac failure. Inter-mittent courses of diphosphonate or calcitonin usually provide good symptomatic benefit when pain is present.

Overgrowth and deformity of Pagetic bone at the base of the skull can lead to brainstem compression. Deafness may be caused by compression of the eighth cranial nerve, or through involvement of the ossicles of the inner ear.

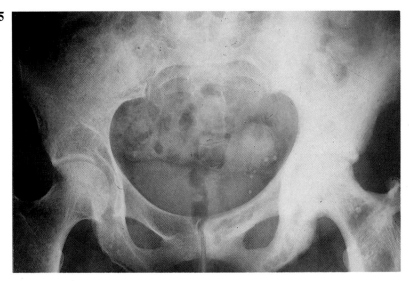
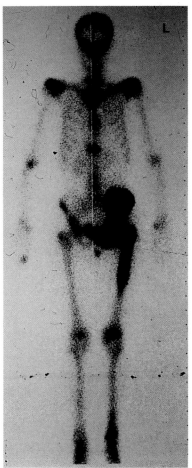

295 & 296 Asymptomatic Paget's disease of the pelvis. This female patient was first found to have raised SAP upon blood screening. X-ray of the pelvis (the most commonly affected area) revealed the typical changes of Paget's disease (**295**). The bone scan (**296**) confirmed the involvement of the left hemipelvis, left upper femur and an isolated lower thoracic vertebra. She remained asymptomatic 6 years later (at which point, treatment had still not been necessary) and the SAP level was around twice the upper limit of normal. If sudden pain were to develop, it might indicate involvement of the hip joint, or rarely, the development of a sarcoma.

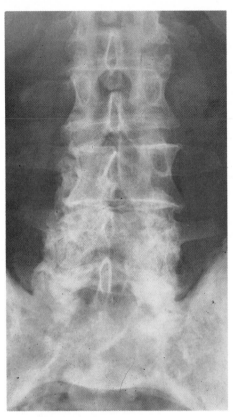

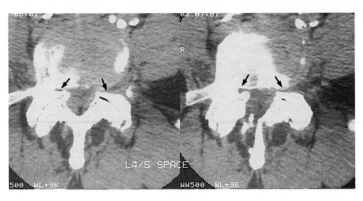

297 & 298 Paget's disease of the spine. This 65-year-old man first presented with claudication. The pain was unilateral, associated with paraesthesia, and in an L5 distribution. On the X-ray (**297**), L4 demonstrates patchy sclerosis and is enlarged; the enlargement is typical of Paget's disease and makes a sclerotic bony secondary unlikely. There was also a grade 2 spondylolisthesis of L4 on L5 (*see* **171**) on the lateral view. The CT scan (**298**) shows the patchy Pagetic changes in L4, affecting the body and the posterior elements of the vertebra. The latter are impinging on the lateral recesses, narrowing the exit foramina, which are already constricted by the spondylolisthesis. This caused nerve root impingement. (The SAP was 3 times the upper limit of normal, but the acid phosphatase was normal.) Despite the spondylolisthesis, his leg pain responded well to a 2-month course of calcitonin, and he remained pain-free 5 years later, although his SAP was still slightly raised.

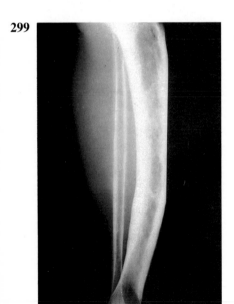

299 Bowing of the tibia in Paget's disease. Pagetic bone is softer than normal, and bony enlargement, together with anterior bowing of the tibia, occasionally leads to this typical deformity. Denser bone is deposited on the concave side, and painful fracture lines at right angles to the cortex may occur on the convex side. Lateral bowing of the femur can also arise, and an affected femoral neck may fracture.

Hypermobility syndrome

The normal range of movement of any joint is determined by its anatomy, but it also varies according to the relative laxity of the surrounding soft tissues. This laxity differs between races and individuals. It decreases with age and is increased in Ehlers–Danlos syndrome and Marfan's disease, in both of which, abnormal collagen is present in the connective tissue. Joint hypermobility may be localised (hyperextension of the knee is common is West Indians, and hyperextension of the fingers in people from the Indian subcontinent) or generalised. It is useful to dancers, gymnasts and some athletes, and may, to a certain extent, be acquired by practice. The combination of increased joint laxity and untrained muscles may lead, however, to joint and spinal pain and a raised incidence of secondary degenerative joint and spinal changes. Regular exercises to strengthen the muscles and stabilise the joints and spine are helpful in controlling pain and delaying deterioration. It is important to explain to the patient that the syndrome rarely leads to severe chronic pain or to functional impairment

Generalised hypermobility is defined by the following features in a Caucasian:
- Hyperextension of the little fingers of more than 90°.
- Ability to bend the thumbs backwards to touch the forearm (**300**).
- Hyperextension of the elbow beyond 10°.
- Ability to place the hands flat to the floor, standing with straight knees (**301**).
- Ability to flex the hip beyond 90° with a straightened leg.
- Hyperextension of the knees beyond 10°.

300

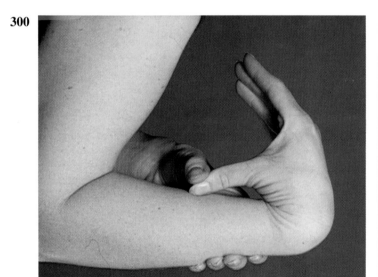

301

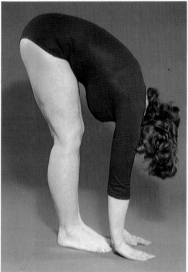

300 & 301 Hypermobility syndrome.

Polymyalgia rheumatica (PMR) and giant cell arteritis

PMR is a relatively common disease, occurring mainly in patients over 60 years of age, and increasing in frequency with advancing age. It causes severe pain and stiffness of the limb girdles. The pain and stiffness are typically worse for several hours in the morning and resolve later in the day, only to recur the next morning. There may also be weight loss, night sweats, depression and a raised serum hepatic alkaline phosphatase. Proximal synovial joints may be inflamed. The disease is diagnosed by its typical clinical picture, the presence of a raised ESR, and the exclusion of other possible causes including RA (*see* Chapter 1), carcinomatous myopathy, infective endocarditis and polymyositis (*see* p.104). RA may present with a polymyalgic picture in the elderly, the diagnosis only becoming apparent as the dose of steroids is reduced and the chronic joint involvement emerges.

Starting with a single daily dose of 10–15 mg in the morning, treatment with prednisolone is dramatically effective. The dose should be reduced very slowly (by no more than 1 mg every month) to prevent recurrence. The rate of reduction should be modified, however, according to the symptoms and the ESR, and may have to be halted or reversed. In about 75% of cases, treatment can be discontinued completely within 12–24 months, but some patients require a single daily dose of 2–5 mg prednisolone for longer. Preventive measures against osteoporosis should be considered in these patients (*see* p.131).

Temporal arteritis (TA)

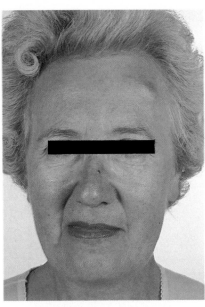
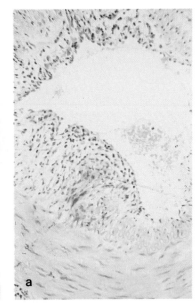
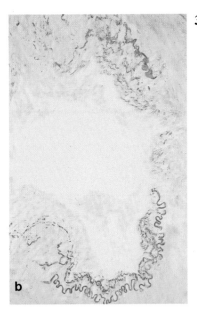

a

b

302 & 303(a) & (b) Temporal arteritis. It is important to recognise PMR, not only because the distressing symptoms can be readily controlled, but also because of its association with giant cell arteritis. The two diseases may present separately or, rarely, at the same time. The symptoms of TA are of malaise and fever with severe, usually unilateral, headache and scalp tenderness. Claudication of the jaw may produce facial pain when chewing. The temporal artery is typically tender, swollen and pulseless, but may be clinically normal. In severe cases the swollen and red temporal artery may be visible on the affected side. The use of corticosteroids (but not of NSAIDs) in PMR reduces the risk of developing TA, but the patient should be warned to report any sudden onset of severe headache and scalp tenderness urgently, because it may indicate the development of TA and a risk of sudden blindness due to involvement of the central retinal arteries.

The ESR is raised, often to above 50 mm in the first hour.

Diagnosis is confirmed by finding this typical picture of intimal thickening, giant cells and disruption of the internal elastic lamina (best seen on the elastin stain, **303(b)**) in the temporal artery. The biopsy should be performed before or within 24 hours of starting treatment with high doses of prednisolone (60 mg per day), and examined carefully, as the appearances may occur only patchily along its length. The dose of prednisolone can be reduced gradually over a few weeks to 20 mg daily as a single dose in the morning, but the reduction should be much slower thereafter. Any recurrence of headache should be treated with an increased dose, but care should to be taken to confirm that the headaches are due to temporal arteritis (a raised ESR is indicative) and not to muscle contraction headaches, brought on by understandable anxiety about the risk of visual loss.

For a discussion of other types of arteritis, *see* pp.108–111.

Behçet's disease

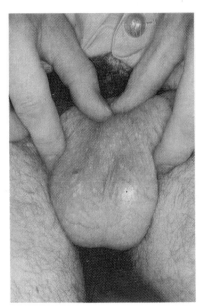

304 Scrotal ulceration in Behçet's disease. Behçet's disease is rare and of unknown aetiology. It more commonly presents in young males, with a triad of recurrent painful oral and genital ulceration, and iritis. There are striking geographical variations in its prevalence, it being more common in the Middle East and in Japan. About 60% of cases also develop an episodic or chronic arthritis. The knee is affected in most patients, but an asymmetrical polyarticular arthritis is usual. Other clinical features include: erythema nodosum (*see* **305**); superficial thrombophlebitis; retinal vasculitis or optic neuritis, which may result in blindness; and a variety of neurological problems, for example, meningitis, stroke and cerebellar syndromes. Optic and cerebral involvement are both potentially serious and warrant treatment with corticosteroids. Colchicine may help the orogenital ulceration and arthritis. Specialist care is essential.

Erythema nodosum

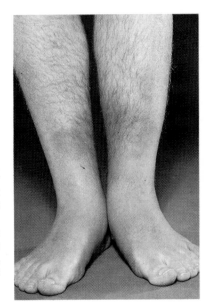

305 Erythema nodosum. The patient complains primarily of tender, red, subcutaneous nodules, principally on the shins, which typically bruise as they fade, but never ulcerate. They settle spontaneously over a few days or weeks, but may recur. Around 60–70% of patients develop arthralgia or arthritis, most often of the ankles and knees.

The most common cause of erythema nodosum is sarcoidosis (*see* below). In such cases a chest X-ray may show bilateral hilar lymphadenopathy. Other causes include a variety of infections, drug sensitivities, inflammatory bowel disease and, occasionally, malignancy. In 10% of patients, no cause is found. Treatment is with rest, NSAIDs or, in a few cases, a short course of corticosteroids.

Sarcoidosis

The most common presenting features of sarcoidosis are fever, malaise, cough or erythema nodosum (*see also* **305**). Bilateral hilar lymphadenopathy is usually demonstrable on chest X-rays. An associated symmetrical inflammatory arthritis, usually of the knees, ankles and hands, is not uncommon, particularly when erythema nodosum is present. The arthritis generally resolves within 1–3 months and does not lead to joint destruction. In some cases it follows a relapsing course. Iridocyclitis may also occur and cause confusion with a seronegative spondarthritis, but there is no association with sacroiliitis or HLA B27. Treatment of the acute arthritis is with NSAIDs, or with steroids if they are indicated for other reasons, such as hypercalcaemia or severe eye involvement.

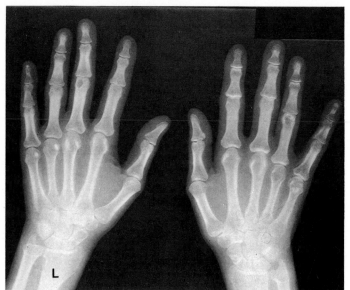

306 Chronic bone sarcoidosis. Chronic sarcoidosis may occasionally be associated with the formation of bone lesions, which appear on X-rays as sharply circumscribed lytic areas in the bones of the hands (left middle proximal phalanx) and feet. These lesions are usually asymptomatic. Chronic cutaneous sarcoidosis may coexist.

Neuropathic arthritis (Charcot's joints)

307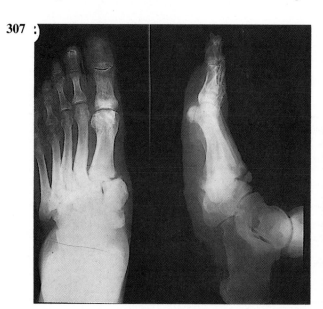

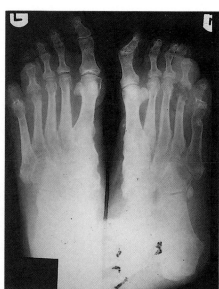 **308**

307 & 308 Neuropathic diabetic foot. (Peripheral neuropathy in diabetes mellitus leads to impaired pain perception in some. This may lead to chronic ulceration caused by trauma and, sometimes, to underlying destruction of bone and resultant deformity. In **307** the midtarsal region has collapsed, producing a 'rocker-bottom' foot. Osteomyelitis, which is a major risk due to secondary infection from skin ulceration, has caused severe damage to the lateral metatarsal of the right foot in **308**. Expert chiropody, carefully made surgical shoes and good general foot care are essential preventive measures, which also go some way towards dealing with such problems once they have arisen. Surgery may be necessary as a final resort.

A variety of neurological conditions which involve loss of proprioception and/or deep pain sensation may lead to severe joint destruction. Increased trauma and stress to the desensitised joint during motion are thought to be the main causes, eventually resulting in cartilage loss, repeated subchondral fractures and marked periarticular new bone formation. Onset is insidious and usually involves one joint, although others become affected in a distribution that reflects the primary neurological disturbance: knees, hips, ankles and lumbar spine in tabes dorsalis; the small joints of the feet in diabetic neuropathy; and the shoulders, elbows and cervical spine in syringomyelia. Rarer causes include peripheral nerve injury, lepromatous neuropathy, and peroneal muscular atrophy. Treatment is aimed at stabilising the joint with braces, although these may produce pressure ulcers, or surgically. Success rates, however, are low

309 Tabes dorsalis. There is early destruction of the left knee, mimicking OA. The right knee reveals more typical advanced changes, with large, disorganised osteophytes and fragmentation of the lateral tibial plateau.

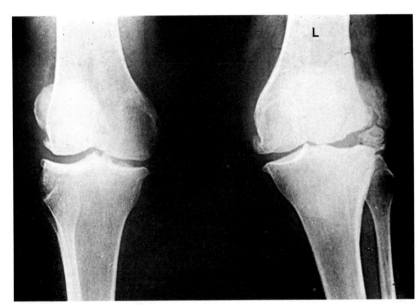

309

310 Advanced tabetic neuropathic arthritis of the hips. The gross destruction and massive, bizarrely distributed new bone formation around the joint are typical. As in all such cases of neuropathic joints, the discomfort is mild in relation to the gross radiological changes.

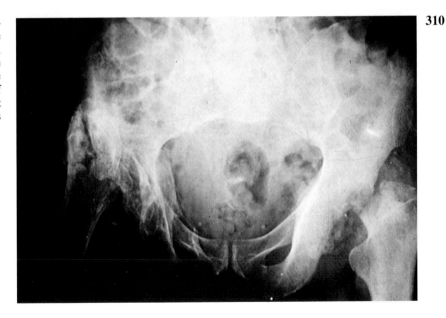

310

Hypertrophic (pulmonary) osteoarthropathy (HPOA)

HPOA is an unusual condition, which presents with persistent pain and tenderness of the hands, feet or distal long bones. Generally, there is an associated arthritis of the fingers, wrists, ankles and knees. The patient usually develops clubbing of fingers and toes, but HPOA may predate the clubbing, occasionally occurring without it. The diagnosis is confirmed radiologically, and requires further investigation for an intrathoracic lesion (most commonly a bronchial carcinoma or pleural tumour, or, rarely, secondary lung deposits).

Chronic suppurative lung diseases, such as lung abscess, chronic bronchiectasis or empyema, are uncommon in developed countries, but can lead to a picture like that seen in HPOA, as can chronic inflammatory bowel disease or biliary cirrhosis. A similar clinical picture may occasionally complicate autoimmune thyroiditis (Graves' disease) (*see* p.130). Patients with established cyanotic heart disease develop HPOA, which reverses if the cardiac shunt is corrected. Regression of the abnormalities is also seen if the primary lung lesion can be removed. The cause is not known, but some cases are hereditary. The periosteum becomes hyperaemic, oedematous and mildly inflamed, as do the synovial membranes of affected joints and the soft tissues of the clubbed digits.

311

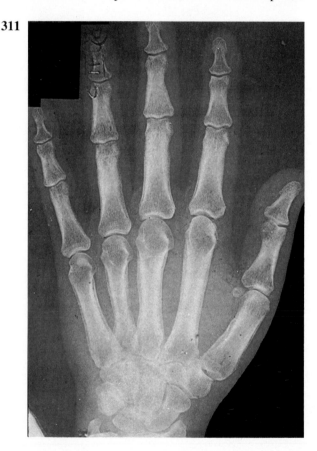

311 HPOA of the hand. There is a line of periosteal new bone formation along the metacarpals and proximal phalanges in this well-established case, but less marked changes are easily missed. Similar alterations may also be seen in the distal radius and ulna and in the feet and lower legs. When the primary cause cannot be reversed, treatment is symptomatic, using NSAIDs where necessary.

Aseptic necrosis of bone

A number of conditions are associated with occasional vascular impairment without local infection, leading to the development of areas of bone infarction or to aseptic necrosis. Causes include fracture of the femoral neck, inflammatory arthritis, SLE, caisson disease (affecting divers who undergo decompression that is too rapid) and sickle-cell disease (*see* p.125). It is also associated with high-dose corticosteroid treatment. Around 30% of cases are idiopathic, however. The femoral head, the humeral head, and the talus are the most commonly affected sites. Symptoms depend upon the site, but pain is often severe, requiring rest and analgesia. The resultant bone damage is generally treatable only by surgical means.

312 Aseptic necrosis of the hip.
This elderly patient developed acute hip pain 2 years after receiving high doses of steroids for 3 months, for ulcerative colitis. The X-ray shows a discrete area of bone sclerosis and collapse in the femoral head. The other hip became affected 6 months later. Bilateral hip replacement restored normal mobility.

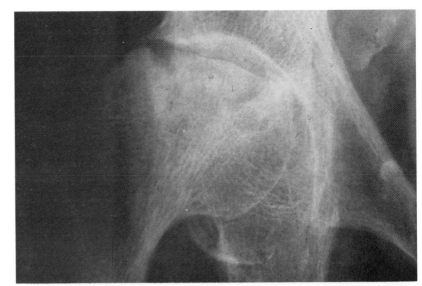

313 Aseptic necrosis of the humeral head. This patient presented with severe shoulder pain; his employment as a deep sea diver provided the clue, and the X-ray shows a well-defined area of sclerosis in the head of the humerus. The acute pain settled, but he developed secondary osteoarthritis, eventually requiring total shoulder arthroplasty.

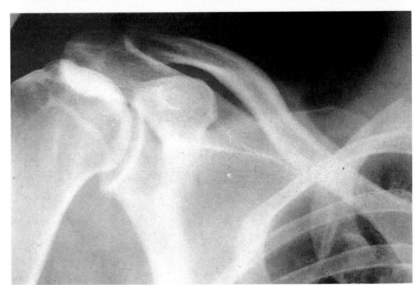

314 MRI of early aseptic necrosis of the hip. Although X-rays clearly demonstrate the abnormality once it has become established, they are normal during the first few weeks. MRI is now the most sensitive early means of demonstrating aseptic necrosis. This patient has bilateral changes, with a dense irregular sclerotic line in both femoral heads and irregularity of the articular surfaces. If MRI is not available, an isotope bone scan will also prove positive before X-ray changes are apparent.

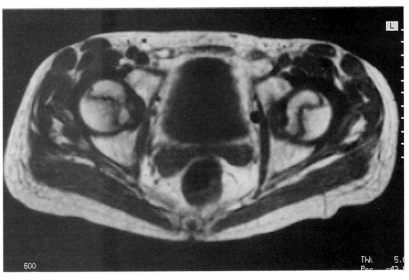

Myelomatosis

Myelomatosis is caused by a malignant plasmacytoma. It usually presents with anaemia, malaise or frank bone marrow suppression by the malignant plasma cell clone, but may also manifest as pain due to rib or vertebral fractures resulting from myeloma deposits. The diagnosis is confirmed by the detection of free immuno-globulin light chains (Bence-Jones protein) in the urine, and a myeloma (M) band on the serum electrophoretic strip. A bony deposit near a joint, usually the hip, may lead to an acute monarthritis. Treatment is with analgesia and local radiotherapy, followed by intermittent chemotherapy.

315

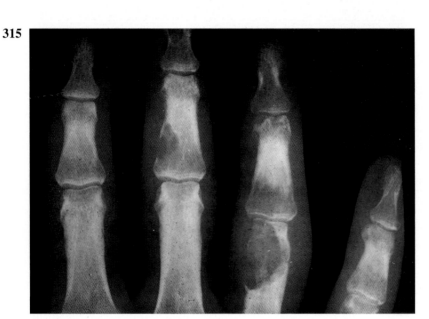

315 Amyloid deposits in the phalanges. A symmetrical peripheral polyarthritis which mimics RA may occur in myelomatosis. X-rays reveal destructive lesions in the bone adjacent to affected joints. These are due to amyloid deposits. The amyloid protein is derived from the light chains of immunoglobulins – amyloid AL protein (*see also* p.46).

Haemochromatosis

316

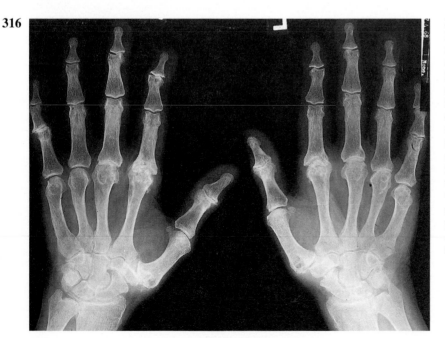

316 The hand of a patient with haemochromatosis. Haemochromatosis is a disorder of iron metabolism and storage, which may be hereditary or acquired. In patients over the age of 50 years, there is an increased incidence of chondrocalcinosis (*see* p.64), even if the iron overload has been successfully treated. The pattern of chondrocalcinosis and arthritis is unusual, frequently affecting the second and third metacarpophalangeal joints, wrists, knees and hips. Progressive cartilage loss, sclerosis, and osteophyte and cyst formation occur. Acute pseudogout (*see* **154**) may develop.

Arthritis in familial Mediterranean fever (FMF)

FMF is common in individuals from the eastern Mediterranean region, but it can occur in those of other origins. It is inherited as an autosomal recessive disease of unknown cause, and first presents in teenagers or young adults as recurrent episodes of fever, pleurisy or peritonitis. Most attacks last 1–3 days and may be very severe. Two-thirds of patients have arthralgia or frank arthritis, commonly of the knee during the attacks. Joints are rarely permanently damaged. Amyloid of the AA type (*see* p.46) is an important cause of long-term morbidity and of mortality, and usually first presents as proteinuria. The diagnosis of FMF is clinical and by exclusion of other causes; the family history or origin of the patient may be helpful clues. Treatment with intermittent or long-term colchicine reduces the severity and frequency of attacks.

Disorders of lipid metabolism and lipid storage diseases

Patients with familial dysbetalipoproteinaemia may suffer episodic attacks of a migratory arthritis of unknown cause.

317

318

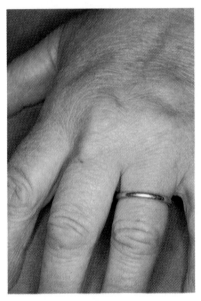
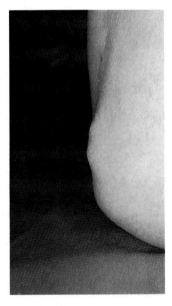

317 & 318 Tendon xanthomata in familial hypercholesterolaemia. This patient has tendon xanthomata on the extensor tendon of the middle finger (**317**) and on the elbow (**318**), which superficially resemble rheumatoid nodules (*see* **28 & 29**). The presence of xanthelasmata around the eyes provides a clue to the diagnosis of this lipid disorder, which is confirmed by finding raised fasting blood cholesterol levels. In view of the increased risk of coronary heart disease, patients will require dietary advice and treatment.

319

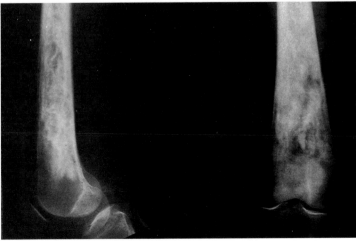

319 Gaucher's disease. This rare autosomal recessive disorder is the most common of a series of lysosomal storage diseases. In the adult form, hepatosplenomegaly, pneumonia and bone pain frequently arise. A distinctive storage cell appears in the bone marrow, and extensive lytic lesions are found in the long bones.

Reflex sympathetic dystrophy

Reflex sympathetic dystrophy may follow trauma, surgery or a stroke. The ankle and foot, or the wrist and hand are most commonly affected, although the whole limb may be involved. After a delay of several days or weeks, the patient develops burning pain, hyperaesthesia, stiffness and puffiness of the affected part. The skin becomes reddened, smooth and glossy. Local temperature changes and increased sweating may occur. The pain is invariably out of proportion to the preceding injury and is the predominant feature in most. A later dystrophic phase develops in some, and the affected part becomes cold and purple. The cause is unknown, but it involves sensitisation of nociceptive mechanisms with consequently heightened pain perception and an increase in sympathetic efferent activity. Recovery is generally spontaneous, but it is accelerated by adequate pain relief, together with movement of the affected joints despite the pain. In about 50% of severe cases, a guanethidine block of the affected limb produces good results.

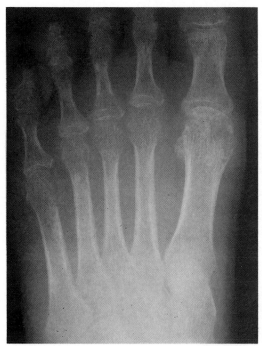

320

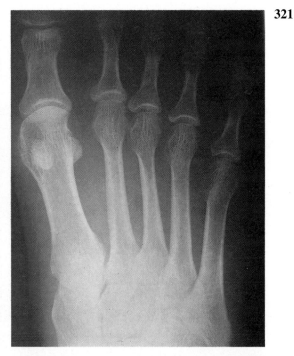

321

320–322 X-rays and a bone scan of patients with reflex sympathetic dystrophy. Radiologically, there is obvious patchy osteopenia of the foot or hand. This is also seen on bone scan as patchy increase of uptake, which is not localised to the joints. **320 & 321** demonstrate the feet of a woman who had experienced severe pain following a minor injury to the left ankle. There is striking generalised patchy osteopenia of the affected foot (**320**), in contrast with the unaffected side (**321**), and the foot itself was puffy and shiny. The bone scan (**322**) is of a different patient who had suffered a cerebrovascular accident several weeks prior to developing a painful shoulder, together with pain and swelling of the hand. The scan (**322**) demonstrates the patchy uptake of isotope in this condition. A similar picture may occur in some patients with acute shoulder pain (shoulder–hand syndrome). Pain and patchy osteoporosis, with or without the skin changes, may occur around the knee, and is known as disuse osteoporosis.

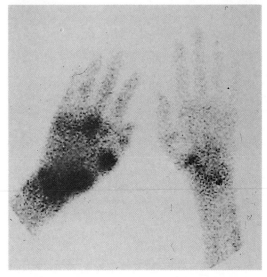

322

10 Soft-tissue rheumatism and local injection techniques

Local corticosteroid injections for soft-tissue lesions, and intra-articular injections for arthritis, are important items in the rheumatologist's armamentarium. The procedures are safe, provided that a few basic rules are followed and scrupulous care is taken to avoid introducing infection. A sound knowledge of basic anatomy is required, and the injections are best performed under supervision on the first few occasions.

Potential complications

The most common complication is a brief postinjection flare of pain, which may be associated with a brisk inflammatory reaction and last for up to 48 hours. It is thought that the flare is caused by the microcrystalline formulation of the corticosteroids, although it is not clear why they do not themselves suppress the inflammation. It is best to forewarn patients that this painful flare may occur, so that they are not worried by it and can plan to rest after the injection if necessary.

If the injection is made superficially, either into soft tissue or into a small joint, it may, very occasionally, produce a small area of skin depigmentation at the injection site, and/or some subcutaneous fat atrophy. The latter may lead to long-term, occasionally permanent, scarring. Again, it is best to forewarn the patient of these possibilities.

Infection is seldom introduced at the time of the procedure as long as the basic precautions described below (*see* 'General aspects of local injection techniques') are scrupulously observed. Nonetheless, any fluid aspirated should always be sent for bacterial culture, and arrangements must be made for the result to be checked.

The most serious complication arises when corticosteroid is injected into an infected joint. This may lead to catastrophic local damage to the joint. Most previously fit patients who develop an infected joint are febrile and very ill, and the joint is extremely painful, hot and inflamed, and thus easily diagnosed. However, in a patient with RA (particularly one taking corticosteroids by mouth), or in an immunocompromised or elderly patient, these systemic features of infection and the extreme local pain and inflammation may be absent. It is in such patients that the risk of inadvertent introduction of steroid into an already infected joint are greatest.

If in doubt:

- *Aspirate the fluid and send it for culture and sensitivity testing.*
- *Refer the patient urgently for specialist advice.*
- *Do not inject steroid.*
- *Do not start antibiotics without first obtaining synovial fluid and blood for culture.*
  An infected joint is a medical emergency.

If clinically indicated, antibiotics should be started immediately (*see also* **64 & 65**). If the culture is unexpectedly positive and steroid has already been injected, the patient should be admitted urgently, further cultures taken and antibiotic treatment commenced.

General aspects of local injection techniques

Local injections should be performed carefully using a no-touch technique. Scrupulous cleansing of the patient's skin with chlorhexidine and thorough hand washing are essential. Provided that great care is taken, it is not essential to use gloves and a gown, unless there is a risk that the patient is hepatitis B- or HIV-positive.

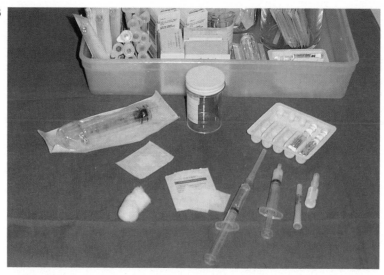

323 Equipment needed for joint aspiration and injection. The equipment for the injection should include cleansing material, swabs and a dressing, syringes of local anaesthetic and the steroid preparation chosen, empty syringes for aspiration and a sterile container into which any aspirated fluid can be placed. Everything must be easily to hand.

The following points should be observed:

- The patient should be sitting or lying comfortably in a quiet room, on a couch set at the correct height for the operator.

- Palpate the area to be injected and then mark and clean the site carefully. Any further palpation should be conducted through a sterile swab or wearing sterile gloves.

- Use a clean needle which has not been used to draw up the local anaesthetic and corticosteroid.

- Without touching the needle, warn the patient that the initial prick will hurt and that the local anaesthetic will sting. However skilled you may become, use local anaesthetic as the needle is slowly advanced.

- As the needle is advanced, repeatedly attempt to aspirate any fluid. Once fluid is obtained, change the syringe and aspirate fully. Examine the aspirate macroscopically. If it is purulent or an infected lesion is suspected, send it for culture and do not inject any steroid. If it is clear or only slightly cloudy and you are confident that is is not infected, change the syringe to that containing the steroid and inject it slowly

- If the injection is to be made into a soft-tissue lesion, once you judge the needle to be in the correct position, change the syringe and inject the steroid.

- Cover the injection site with an adhesive dressing. Advise the patient about rest which is appropriate to the procedure concerned.

Specific lesions and injection techniques

Lesions around the elbow

324 & 325 Lateral epicondylitis (tennis elbow). The patient with tennis elbow complains of pain at the lateral epicondyle, which often radiates to the extensor muscles of the forearm. The pain is increased by gripping or squeezing, especially when the elbow is straight and the wrist dorsiflexed – the power grip position. There is often very localised tenderness either over the epicondyle itself or over the radiohumeral joint. The tender spot should be injected with 1 ml of a corticosteroid, which should be directed onto the surface of the bone at the tendinous insertion. Use local anaesthetic both to introduce the needle and to anaesthetise the periostium, which is usually very sensitive. Warn the patient that the pain may increase considerably for several days and tell them to rest the arm until it is clear that the pain is receding. In recurrent cases it may be necessary to follow a second injection with physiotherapy (ultrasound and stretching exercises).

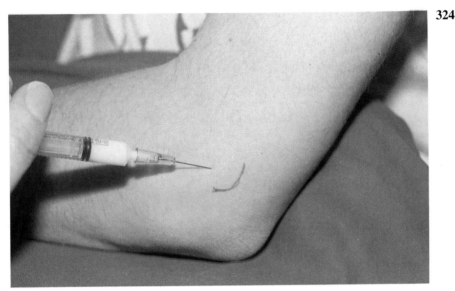

324

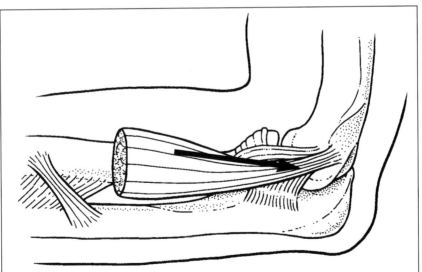

325

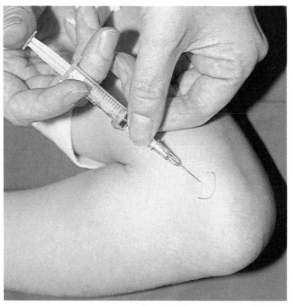 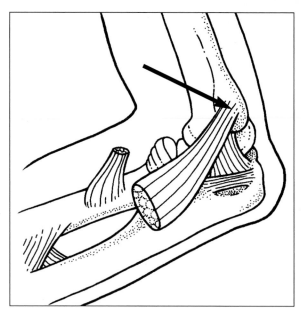

326 & 327 Medial epicondylitis (golfer's elbow). In golfer's elbow the pain is felt over the medial epicondyle and the wrist flexors in the proximal forearm, especially when the fingers are gripping, with the wrist locked in flexion. Carrying a loaded tea tray, for example, becomes painful. The procedure is the same as that for tennis elbow, but care should be taken to ensure that the ulnar nerve is not injured by approaching the lesion from the antecubital side. The injection is most easily performed while the patient lies supine, with the hand behind the neck and the elbow out to the side.

Lesions around the shoulder

328

329

330

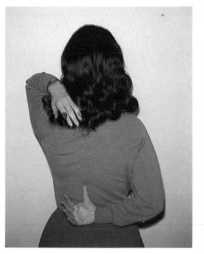 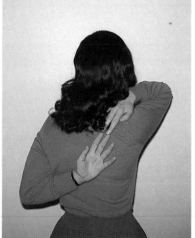 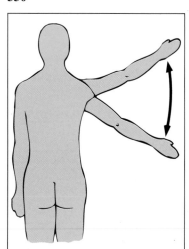

328–330 Painful lesions of the rotator cuff of the shoulder – painful arc syndrome. The painful arc syndrome is one of the most common rheumatological problems. Patients complain of severe pain in the upper arm, which is generally worse just below the tip of the shoulder. If severe, the pain radiates to the rest of the upper arm and, occasionally, to the thumb. It is never associated with paraesthesia, a feature which helps to distinguish it from a C6 nerve root lesion (*see* p.70). The pain is frequently very severe at night, although this is true of a painful shoulder whatever the cause, and patients feel unable to lie on the affected side. They will have noted either that the shoulder is restricted or that it hurts to elevate it or to reach up and backwards. Putting the arm into a coat sleeve is often painful. The neck may be mildly painful on the affected side. This is generally caused by painful muscle spasm as a painful shoulder is often held elevated and the arm adducted, both in order to protect it and to reduce pain. Neck movements are only slightly restricted, if at all, and rarely painful.

On examination, there may be wasting of the supra- and/or infraspinatus muscles if the problem is long-standing. If the arm is not so painful that it is held immobilised, it may be possible passively to raise the arm to full elevation. The patient is then asked to actively lower it sideways. Pain generally occurs, or is exacerbated, during the middle of the range (60–120°) (**330**) and can cause an obvious break in the normally smooth downwards movement of the arm. Specific pain on active internal or external rotation, or abduction against resistance, may help to localise the lesion to the relevant muscle tendon and, thus, to the anterior or posterior aspect of the rotator cuff.

This patient demonstrates marked restriction of internal rotation in extension (reaching behind the back) of the right shoulder (**327**), although there is no restriction when reaching behind the neck with the right arm (**328**). The left shoulder is unaffected.

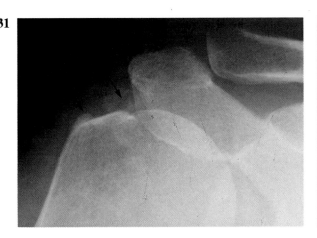

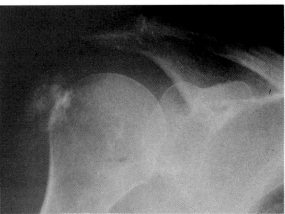

331 & 332 Calcific tendinitis and bursitis. It is not necessary to X-ray a painful shoulder unless the case is atypical or the pain persists. In some resistant cases (**331**) calcific deposits can be demonstrated (arrows) in the tendon, at the site of inflammation. If the deposits are large, attempts should be made to aspirate them through a wide-bore needle, under X-ray screening. Successful treatment usually leads to

disappearance of the deposits, although they may persist without continuing pain.

In subacromial bursitis the pain is more diffuse and often more severe. It may produce very marked splinting of shoulder movements. The second X-ray (**332**) demonstrates the more diffuse calcification that is typical of subacromial bursitis.

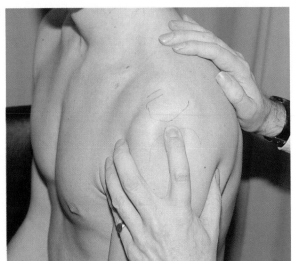

333 Localising the site for a subacromial injection.
Although it is sometimes possible to achieve a more certain effect by directing the injection to that part of the rotator cuff deemed to be specifically affected, the procedure is not easy unless it is performed under direct vision during arthroscopy. A technically easier approach, which is helpful in about 70% of cases, is to direct the steroid into the subacromial bursa.

The groove between the acromion and the head of the humerus is palpated. This is best performed when the patient is seated, with the arm hanging freely beside them. The groove is usually 1–2 cm below the tip of the shoulder. It may be difficult to feel in fat or well-muscled individuals, or in older patients who have a torn rotator cuff (*see* **336**).

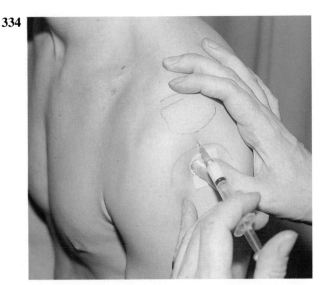

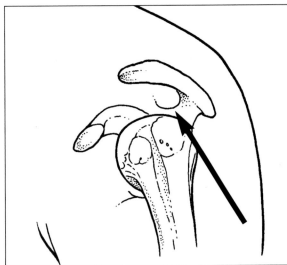

334 & 335 Injection of the subacromial bursa. The bursa is best approached from the side, with the needle directed medially and slightly upwards. The needle is advanced, injecting local anaesthetic. If bone is touched, the needle should be slightly adjusted, up or down. Once the correct route has been found, the needle is inserted deep enough to lie well under the acromion. At this point, it should be possible to inject a couple of millilitres of local anaesthetic with little resistance. An attempt at aspiration should be made, although it is uncommon to obtain fluid unless there is an arthritis or bursitis; 1 ml of the selected corticosteriod is then injected.

One advantage of using a reasonable volume of local anaesthetic is that it will often produce a temporary but marked improvement in the painful arc of movement. This reassures both the patient and the doctor that the injection has been made at the correct site. Once the anaesthetic wears off, a severe flare of the pain occasionally occurs, lasting about 24 hours. The patient should be warned not to use the arm too much in the first week or so, even if the pain improves, in order to avoid a recurrence. In some cases, a second injection may be needed after 3–6 weeks, but no earlier. If the pain resolves but stiffness persists, physiotherapy is helpful.

336 Torn rotator cuff. In the older patient, chronic impingement of the rotator cuff on the under surface of the acromion may lead to eventual rupture of the cuff. This may also occur in an inflammatory arthritis, such as RA (*see* **57**). The tear may develop acutely, causing immediate pain, or painlessly and gradually. The end result is that abduction is seriously restricted. Radiologically, there is often roughening and sclerosis of the greater tuberosity and of the under surface of the acromion. If the problem is painful, a local corticosteroid injection can sometimes provide relief. However, corticosteroids can weaken the cuff, occasionally leading to a cuff tear themselves. The injection technique is similar to that described above, although a more posterior approach makes it easier to introduce the needle between the closely apposed bones. In otherwise fit individuals, or after traumatic rupture in a sportsman, surgical repair is possible.

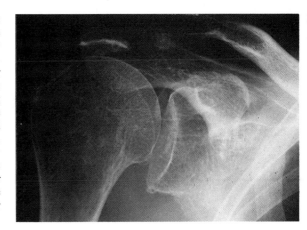

Lesions of the wrist

337 **338**

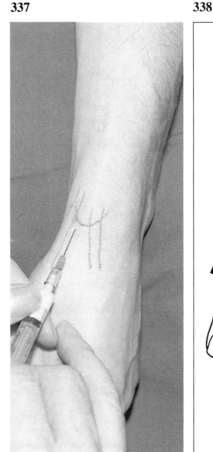

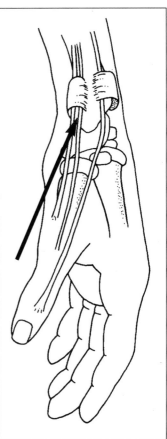

337 & 338 De Quervain's tenosynovitis. De Quervain's tenosynovitis produces pain over the radial styloid and makes gripping and holding things difficult. Local swelling may arise and there is always local tenderness, which may be over the styloid itself, or just proximal or distal to it. Occasionally, both the swelling and the tenderness are marked. The pain can be reproduced over the styloid by forced flexion of the thumb into the palm of the hand. This manoeuvre will also produce pain in first carpometacarpal OA (*see* **124 & 125**), but here the pain is localised more distally, at the tender first CMC joint. De Quervain's tenosynovitis is a common problem in young mothers, developing as their babies grow heavier. It affects the sheath of the tendons of abductor pollicis longus and extensor pollicis brevis as the tendons pass across the radial styloid.

Even if there is no local swelling, the tender tendon sheath and associated tendons can be easily palpated as they pass over the radial styloid. A small needle should be introduced alongside the tendons, using local anaesthetic, and 1 ml of the chosen corticosteroid is then injected; it should not be injected under pressure, as this may indicate injection into the tendon itself. It is usually possible to feel and see the injection filling out the tendon sheath proximally. The local anaesthetic produces a reassuring, if temporary, reduction of the pain. Generally, the steroid takes about 5 days to work. Rarely, a stenosing tenosynovitis occurs, necessitating surgical decompression.

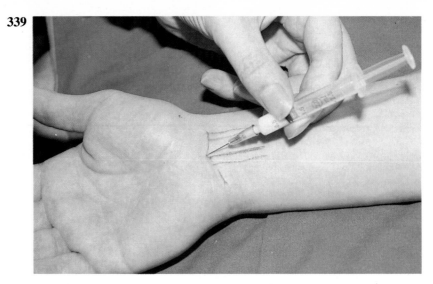

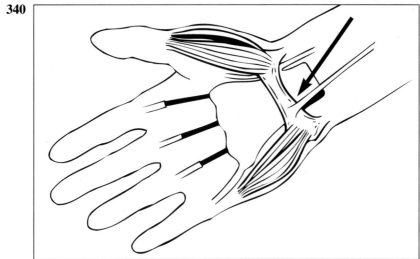

339 & 340 Carpal tunnel syndrome. The typical symptoms are described elsewhere (*see* **106 & 107**). When a resting splint (worn at night) has produced only temporary relief, and when there is no clinical evidence of thenar muscle wasting or of permanent numbness, a local steroid injection into the carpal tunnel will often produce long-term relief. If there is diagnostic doubt, nerve conduction studies should be performed before the injection is undertaken. It is best not to repeat the injection more than once. If improvement does not occur, perform nerve conduction studies to confirm the diagnosis and then refer for surgical decompression.

The carpal tunnel is approached from the direction of the forearm, using a fine needle inserted into the palmar wrist crease just to the ulnar side of the tendon of palmaris longus (if this muscle is present). Local anaesthetic should only be used superficially, as its injection around the nerve often causes prolonged and painful paraesthesia. The syringe is then exchanged for one containing the steroid. A small volume is injected under low pressure – increased pressure suggests that the needle is too superficial or in a tendon and that its position needs adjusting. If this initial low-pressure injection produces immediate pain or paraesthesia in the median nerve distribution, it should be assumed that the needle is in the nerve and needs to be repositioned. Once the correct position is achieved, the entire 1 ml of corticosteroid should be injected *slowly*. This may produce the symptoms of carpal tunnel syndrome towards the end of the procedure. The patients should rest the wrist in a splint for a few days afterwards.

Lesions of the knee

341 Procedure for aspiration and injection of the knee joint. (The detection of an effusion in the knee is described on p.26.) The procedure for aspiration of a knee effusion is simple, once seen and practised a few times. The patient must be resting comfortably, with the leg relaxed and the knee straight. If there is a fixed flexion deformity, it should be supported by a rolled towel. It is easier if the leg is slightly externally rotated. Read the general guidance for intra-articular aspiration and injection before carrying out the procedure (*see* p.145).

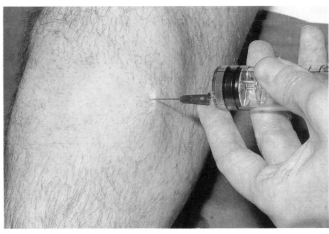

The easiest approach is from the medial side of the knee, around the mid point of the patella. When an effusion is present, there is usually some widening of the gap between the posterior aspect of the patella and the medial femoral condyle. This gap can be further widened by gentle pressure on the suprapatellar pouch (from the nondominant hand or an assistant), displacing the effusion into the main joint. The gap is increased even more by gentle backwards pressure on the lateral border of the patella. The groove should be palpated, and gently marked with a finger nail. The skin can then be carefully cleansed. If further palpation is necessary, it should be performed through a sterile swab, with the nondominant hand. Always use local anaesthetic, injecting a little at a time as the needle is advanced, until a slight increase in resistance is felt – the joint capsule. In cases of acute effusion the capsule may be quite thin and difficult to sense, but in chronic synovitis it may be very tough to penetrate; the toughened capsule can be distinguished from contact with bone (which will feel hard) because it still has a sense of give. Use more local anaesthetic and warn the patient that it may hurt as the needle is advanced through the often sensitive capsule. Once through the capsule, attempt gently to aspirate fluid. If the fluid flows freely and then stops, it is likely that the needle has become blocked either by a synovial frond or by a 'rice' body (a piece of synovium that has become hyalinised and detached). Use a gentle push-and-pull technique and try to drain as much fluid as possible. If a small amount of blood is present, it is probably traumatic in origin and of no significance. A large amount of blood is sometimes present either in a simple haemarthrosis complicating OA, or if the patient has continued to be very active despite the effusion. Its presence does not necessarily alter the plan to instil corticosteroid. If the exudate is inflammatory, the fluid usually appears cloudy or opalescent. If extreme cloudiness or frank pus is seen, the procedure should be terminated, and the fluid sent for urgent Gram staining and culture. *If it is obviously purulent, the patient must be referred immediately to a rheumatologist or orthopaedic surgeon* (*see* p.17).

Once the swelling and pain have settled, the patient should perform graded exercises to restore the power of the quadriceps muscle, which wastes rapidly if a knee swells.

342 Medial ligament of the knee. Sprains of the medial (or lateral) ligaments of the knee may produce local pain at their insertions into the tibia. This is associated with marked local tenderness and pain, which can be reproduced by appropriate medial or lateral stressing of the knee, pulling on the affected tendon. The pain may initially be caused by injury, or arise apparently spontaneously. Medial ligament pain is common in patients who have fat thighs, valgus knees and/or flat feet. The symptoms often occur with mild, probably coincidental, radiological changes of OA of the knee. A local injection of 1 ml of a corticosteroid into the tender area of the surface of the bone, using local anaesthetic to introduce the needle and anaesthetise the periostium, is helpful in some cases. Weight loss should be recommended if appropriate, and medial arch supports may help to prevent recurrences.

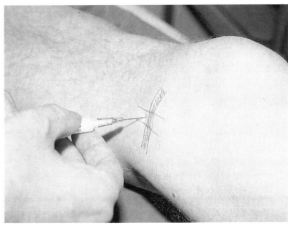

Lesions around the hip

343 Injection of trochanteric bursitis. The pain of trochanteric bursitis is localised to the outer thigh, being most marked over the trochanter itself. The patient will often assume, incorrectly, that it is coming from the hip joint. The pain is aggravated by walking, particularly up and down stairs, and by lying on the affected side. (The distribution of pain is similar to that seen in **meralgia paraesthetica**, which results from compression of the lateral cutaneous nerve of the thigh as it emerges through the fascia lata. However, the latter syndrome is clearly distinguished by the symptoms of painful paraesthesia and numbness that it produces over the anterolateral thigh: such sensory changes are not present in trochanteric bursitis). On examination, there is localised tenderness over the greater trochanter itself or, sometimes, just proximal to it. Discomfort is usually worsened by active and passive hip movements, but it is the site of the pain that suggests the diagnosis. *Hip joint pain is felt in the groin, buttock and anterior thigh, not over the trochanter or lateral thigh.* The site of maximum tenderness should be injected, using a long needle if the patient is fat. Local anaesthetic and 1 ml of corticosteroid are administered just superficial to the surface of the bone. The patient should rest for a day or so after the procedure, avoiding excessive stair climbing and running for several weeks.

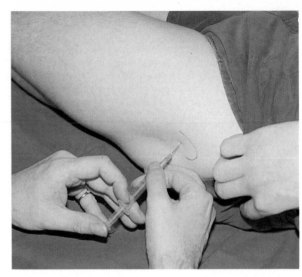

Aspiration and injection of the hip joint is a technically difficult procedure and should be performed by a specialist.

Lesions around the heel

344 Heel pain and injection of plantar fasciitis. Pain under the heel may be associated with a diffuse tenderness of the fibrofatty pad which protects the calcaneum, or with a localised lesion of the insertion of the plantar fascia into the anterior surface of the calcaneum. Both conditions produce pain and tenderness on weight-bearing, but these are more localised in plantar fasciitis. Pain at the insertion of the Achilles tendon into the calcaneum, or over the bursa which lies just proximal to the insertion and anterior to the tendon, is commonly experienced by individuals who have suddenly started either to wear shoes with a lower heel height than usually or to walk barefoot. Problems of this kind often arise on holiday.

All such complaints can be simply helped by asking the patient to wear shoes with thick, shock-absorbing heels, for example, a good pair of trainers, or to insert shock-absorbing pads into the shoes. In cases of plantar fasciitis the heel pad should be cut to a horseshoe shape to relieve pressure on the plantar fascia insertion. If this approach fails, or if the pain is severe, a carefully localised corticosteroid injection can be helpful.

If the pain occurs under the heel, the needle is best inserted from the side, to avoid the very thick skin of the heel pad. Local anaesthetic is essential. The site of maximum tenderness is injected with 1 ml of steroid. Local injection at the site of maximum tenderness will also help painful lesions of the Achilles tendon, but great care must be taken to avoid injecting into the tendon, as this may cause it to rupture. If the pain is in the body of the tendon, a partial tear may be to blame, in which case specialist referral is indicated.

Fibromyalgia (fibrositis syndrome) and related disorders

Patients with fibromyalgia and related disorders (often, but not exclusively, middle-aged and energetic women) can present with an exasperating battery of complaints. To the rheumatologist they complain of **'pain all over'**, to the neurologist of **typical tension headaches**, and to the gastroenterologist of the myriad symptoms of **irritable bowel syndrome**, for example, bloating, diarrhoea and abdominal pain.

Patients with predominantly rheumatological symptoms frequently complain bitterly of long-standing and widespread pain, which has not been helped by the wide variety of drugs and physical techniques that they have already tried. Added to this comes the exasperation of learning that doctors can find nothing wrong on numerous tests, while X-rays reveal minimal OA changes or spondylosis, sometimes (occasionally erroneously) used to dismiss the problem as 'wear and tear'. Patients are often introspective and anxious, but they may have little insight and may be unprepared to concede that anxiety and stress can play a role in the persistence of their symptoms. They are demanding of a doctor's time, expecting consistent explanations for their problems – the rheumatologist's 'heart sink' patient. Although it is of course necessary to exclude serious pathology, the length of time that the symptoms have been present and the patient's ability to carry on despite them are important clues. Indeed, this very drive to continue with a busy life despite the pain is often encouraged by relatives and friends who think of the sufferer as being brave or remarkable. Sleep is usually disturbed and typically unsatisfying, with patients awakening unrefreshed.

345 Trigger points in fibromyalgia. Fibromyalgia is an important and useful diagnosis, which recognises that the one characteristic unifying feature of all these patients is the presence of surprisingly tender and well-defined trigger points. A variety of different points has been described: **345** illustrates the most typical. The exact number and location may be less important than the fact that they all appear in parts of the body that are tender in every normal individual to a certain extent, being markedly so in these patients. The trigger points largely represent areas where muscle or tendon is inserted into bone, so-called 'entheses'. Not only is the finding of these trigger points of diagnostic significance, it also comes as a surprise to many patients, who are then grateful that, at last, something abnormal has been found.

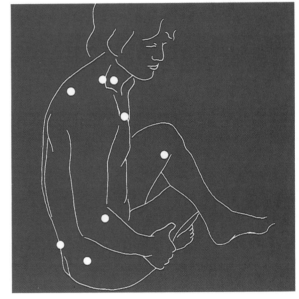

345

The management of these cases is complex and often exhausting. Although reassurance that the pain can be explained and is not due to some fatal or potentially disabling disease is gratefully received, it is usually tempered by the realisation that the syndrome is itself persistent and difficult to relieve; the trigger points are generally over muscular insertions into bone, but are only occasionally helped by local injections. There are no clear descriptions of abnormal pathology, either at these sites or in the muscles. Reflex muscle spasm, increased awareness of normal or slightly increased bodily functions and sensory input, and a pattern of pain which itself induces painful muscle spasm, creating a vicious circle, are all concepts which can be used to explain the syndrome.

There is probably some overlap between fibromyalgia and the **chronic fatigue syndrome** (also known as chronic postviral fatigue syndrome in those who describe a well-defined preceding viral illness). Sufferers complain of extreme and easy fatiguability, to the extent that normal day-to-day activity may become impossible. A positive and patient approach helps a good number to recover, although it may take weeks or months.

Graded exercise programmes and hydrotherapy may be beneficial, particularly if the patient is generally unfit. Relaxation, yoga and massage can also bring relief. Although analgesics and anti-inflammatory drugs are rarely helpful, they can be tried for brief periods in an attempt to break the pain circle. Amitriptylline used at night also helps some patients, probably by restoring a more normal sleep pattern, but also because of its antidepressant effect and its known benefit in chronic pain syndromes. Although the drug can help in cases of depression, if the risk of alienating patients is to be avoided, it should be stressed that it is not being used primarily as an antidepressant.

Sufferers are often undeniably difficult and demanding, but they are genuine, and deserve reassurance and help, despite the limitations of current understanding about both the pathological problem and its control.

11 Surgery and rehabilitation in rheumatic diseases

Nowhere is the need for a good working relationship between a rheumatologist and an orthopaedic surgeon more apparent than in the management of patients with chronic and progressive inflammatory arthritis. Such disorders require the continuing supervision of a rheumatologist who is more experienced than the surgeon in the control of the disease by drugs and other means. The surgeon will occasionally be able to perform prophylactic surgical procedures, such as synovectomy, early in the disease, but will play a vital role in managing the small proportion of patients who later develop severe joint damage and deformity.

Surgery is fundamental in the management of a variety of other disorders which may present first to a rheumatologist: the patient with an acute prolapsed disc that has not responded to conservative management, and those requiring nerve and tendon decompressions, such as carpal tunnel syndrome (*see* **106, 107 & 339**), stenosing de Quervain's tenosynovitis (*see* **337**) or shoulder impingement syndromes (*see* pp.148–151). Surgical help and advice is also essential in the management of joint infections and of malignancies or infections of the spine.

Extensive description of surgical interventions and techniques is beyond the scope of this book, but the general principles of surgical management of chronic arthritis are discussed and a few of the surgical procedures used are described.

Surgery in chronic arthritis – general points

It is especially important for any patient with a chronic and progressive arthritis that the realistic aims, expectations and potential risks of any surgical procedure are explained and discussed frankly. In patients who have RA affecting the hips, knees and hindfeet, for example, a forefoot arthroplasty may do little to reduce their pain or increase their mobility, but may be essential to prevent ulceration (*see* **35**) and thus reduce the risk of later blood-borne infection of a local or distant joint. Replacement of a severely damaged hip or knee will decrease pain in the replaced joint and improve mobility, but the mere fact that the patient is more mobile sometimes causes increased pain in the remaining lower limb joints and/or in the upper limbs because of increased weight-bearing through sticks or crutches. The risk of postoperative or delayed infection in any replaced joint is slight but definite, and may leave the patient worse off than before the surgery. This risk has to be discussed honestly, but without frightening patients, when they are making their decision. The potential benefits offered by the procedures being considered should be carefully balanced against the risks.

In all patients with inflammatory polyarthritis, especially RA, the development of neck instability should be borne in mind as a possible risk factor during anaesthetic intubation for surgery (*see* pp.34–37). Lateral views of the cervical spine in neutral, flexion and extension are obligatory and the anaesthetist should be forewarned. It is often sensible to send the patient to the operating theatre wearing a soft collar as a reminder.

Synovectomy

The role of surgical synovectomy in chronic inflammatory arthritis remains controversial. Many surgeons favour open synovectomy in an inflammatory monarthritis of the knee, or in chronic inflammatory polyarthritis which is generally well-controlled by drugs, but in which one or both knees remain the site of significant synovitis. The procedure is not deemed worthwhile if there is any evidence of cartilage or bony damage on X-rays. Some studies suggest that there is an increased risk of stiffening or infection in the operated knee if it later requires replacement arthroplasty. Arthroscopic synovectomy of the knee is possible, although it is even more difficult to remove all of the inflamed synovium through an arthroscope than it is during an open procedure. The true effect of synovectomy on outcome in the longer term has not been studied sufficiently to be regarded as proven. Indeed, the extremely variable and unpredictable outcome of RA means that such surgical procedures are as difficult to assess in a controlled fashion as are the second-line drugs. Synovectomy has no role in osteoarthritis.

Nonsurgical approaches to single joint inflammatory disease, which might be called chemical synovectomy, include the introduction of intra-articular corticosteroids (*see* p.153) or osmic acid. The latter is favoured in some European countries, although not widely used in the UK or the USA. Radiation synovectomy, using either external irradiation or radioactive isotopes prepared in such a way that they can be injected into the joint, is also employed .

Surgical synovectomy of the wrist joint, as part of a procedure which also excises the ulnar styloid, is helpful to prevent rupture of finger extensor tendons (*see* pp. 21 & 161). Specialist hand surgeons strongly advocate the use of surgical synovectomy of the finger joints and of tendon sheaths early in progressive RA, as a means of preventing later damage and deformity. Hand surgery in cases of chronic arthritis should remain the preserve of a specialist hand surgeon.

Osteotomy

Osteotomy is used, for example, in the correction of an uncomplicated hallux valgus, where removal of the prominent bone from the inner aspect of the first metatarsal head and the overlying adventitious bursa (bunion) reduces the local pressure from shoes, or as a means of adjusting the alignment of weight-bearing joints to shift the weight away from one part of the joint. Thus, in single compartment OA of the knee which is complicated by either a valgus or a varus deformity, wedge osteotomy can be used both to reduce the deformity and to shift the weight-bearing surface to the unaffected compartment. Such a procedure will rarely achieve a permanent reduction of pain and disability, but it may be helpful in deferring the need for hemi- or total joint replacement in an otherwise fit young or middle-aged person. Occasionally, realignment arthroplasty can be used in a similar way to defer the need for total replacement of the hip in younger patients.

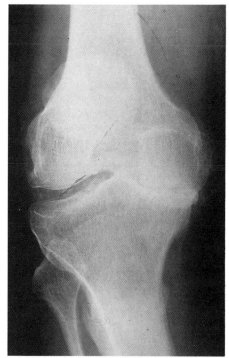 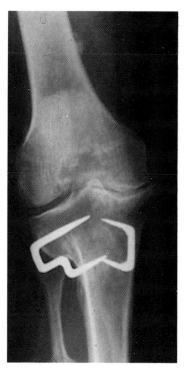

346 & 347 Osteotomy of the knee. This middle-aged but generally fit man had had a medial meniscus excised following a football injury 20 years earlier. Pain in the affected compartment and a deteriorating varus deformity were increasingly limiting mobility. The loss of joint space (on the medial side of the joint in **346**) with early reactive sclerosis and osteophyte formation are typical of OA. An osteotomy was performed, reducing pain and improving mobility for 5 years. The pain in the operated knee remains tolerable despite the advanced changes seen on X-ray (**347**), but increasing pain and instability of the other knee are now the main problem and will require a total knee replacement. (Chondrocalcinosis can be seen in both films – *see* p.64.)

Arthroplasty

Joints can be removed, allowing the formation of a fibrous union (excision arthroplasty), replaced wholly or in part by artificial joints (replacement arthroplasty) or, on occasion, fused (arthrodesis). The procedure undertaken depends in part on the joint involved and in part on the nature of the original problem. In the patient with single joint disease, a total hip or knee replacement may restore virtually normal function, although the patient should be warned of the risk of loosening, and advised not to overstress the new joint; a second replacement of a hip is technically possible, although it is sometimes not as satisfactory as the initial procedure. A second replacement of the knee is more difficult.

In patients with multiple joint disease, excision, replacement or fusion arthroplasty must be planned carefully in the context of the patient as a whole, taking into account the predictable or potential further damage due to progression of the disease, and the state of other joints. Assessment by a rheumatologist and an orthopaedic surgeon in a combined clinic is ideal. Age is an important factor, and youth may count against total joint replacement: the risk of reoperation being required later should be balanced against the likely improvement to the individual's quality of life by the procedure, despite their youth. A young or older patient with multiple damaged joints is less likely to put excessive stress on a replaced joint than is an individual with single joint disease.

The major concern in replacement arthroplasty remains the risk of later blood-borne infection, which may necessitate removal of the artificial joint. A second replacement is sometimes possible once the infected prosthesis has been excised and the infection treated with a prolonged course of antibiotics. Fibrous union may be a satisfactory outcome after removal of an infected replacement, for example, in the elbow and, to a lesser extent, in the hip (a Girdlestone procedure), but an unstable knee is very disabling and requires clumsy splinting to allow weight-bearing, so bony fusion (arthrodesis) is usually attempted. A previously infected joint is less likely to fuse satisfactorily, however, and even if it is successful, a permanently straight knee is itself disabling, particularly when other joints are also damaged.

348   **349**

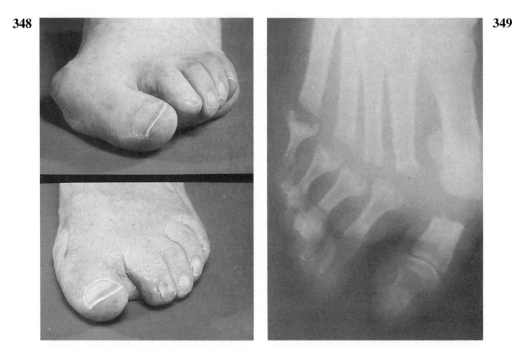

348 & 349 Forefoot excision arthroplasty in a patient with RA. This patient had complained of increasing pain and deformity of the forefeet. Prior to surgery the toes had become hammered and there was a severe hallux valgus. Specially made shoes did not alleviate the pain, and the pressure points began to ulcerate. During the operation the metatarsal heads of the second to fifth toes and the proximal end of the first proximal phalanx were excised, and the head of the first metatarsal head was trimmed. The foot became painless and the ulcerating callosities under the metatarsal heads and over the prominent PIP joints and the painful bunion all resolved.

350–352 Excision and fusion arthroplasty of the wrist. In RA, painful instability of the radioulnar joint at the wrist often leads to dorsal subluxation of the ulnar styloid. The pain may considerably reduce hand function by weakening the power grip and making movements difficult. As shown here (**350**), the roughened end of the dorsally displaced styloid can cause rupture of the wrist extensors (*see also* p.21). Simple excision of the ulnar styloid is often a very effective procedure, during which the inflamed synovium of the wrist and dorsal tendon sheath can be partially excised. This can be used as a preventative procedure to attempt to avoid rupture of the finger extensor tendons.

RA can also severely damage the wrist joint and carpus. In such cases, function may be impaired by severe pain. The use of a splint often improves function and reduces pain, and in some patients the joint fuses spontaneously as a result of the inflammatory process, thereby reducing pain. It is important that the wrist is fused in a slightly dorsiflexed position, the position of optimum function for a power grip. If there is virtually complete loss of dorsiflexion and palmar flexion, with severe pain during any residual movement, surgical fusion of the wrist in slight dorsiflexion is the best option. Here, the preoperative film (**351**) shows exstensive destruction of the wrist joint and proximal carpal bones. In the postoperative film (with the wrist still in a plaster cast) (**352**), the ulnar styloid has been excised and the wrist stabilised by inserting a pin. Replacement arthroplasty of the wrist has been a disappointing procedure to date.

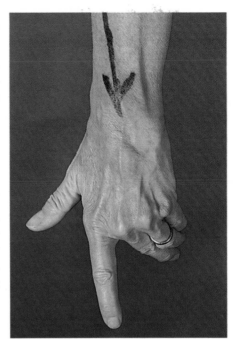

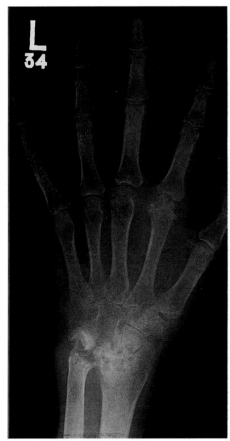

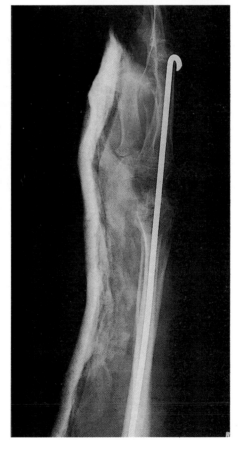

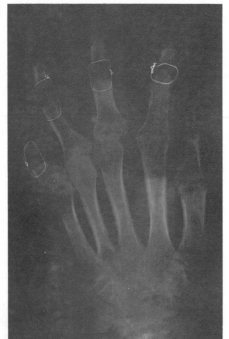

353

353 Arthroplasty of the finger joint. This patient with severe arthritis mutilans and 'telescopic' fingers experienced increasing loss of hand function because of the instability of her PIP joints. Pain in these joints was not a problem, but the decision was made to intervene surgically to improve function. Excision of the joints, together with wiring, produced stable fixed joints and much improved grip and dexterity. Artificial joints can also be inserted into painful PIP or MCP joints, with usually good results. Pain is invariably reduced, but there may be some loss of flexion, which may impair function. For this reason it is important that such surgery is carefully planned, the expected outcome fully explained and the whole process supervised by an experienced hand surgeon. Fusion of the MCP or IP of the thumb may be helpful in restoring pinch grip, if these joints are unstable. DIP joint surgery is rarely necessary or desirable.

354

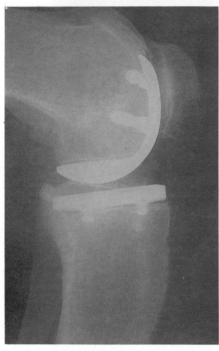

355

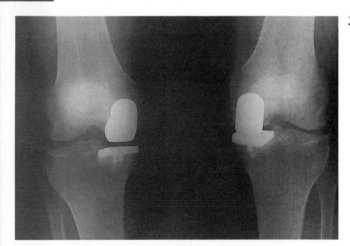

354 & 355 Replacement arthroplasty of the knee. This patient with unicompartmental OA of both knees following earlier excision of the medial menisci underwent bilateral medial compartment hemiarthroplasties. The size of the prosthesis used was carefully selected to reduce the pre-existing moderate varus deformities.

356 Total replacement arthroplasty of the knee.
Severe RA had produced virtually complete loss of cartilage in this knee. On weight-bearing, the pain was severe, as was the varus deformity. A total surface replacement prosthesis has been inserted. These more modern types of knee replacement require less excision of bone than the older models, but depend upon intact medial and lateral collateral ligaments for stability. If joint instability is marked, it may be appropriate to insert a fixed hinge model (not shown) in some patients. Because such fixed hinges do not allow the slight normal rotational movement at the knee during flexion and extension, they are more likely to loosen. In the elderly or severely disabled, who will not place an undue strain on the knee subsequently, such total hinge replacements remain appropriate.

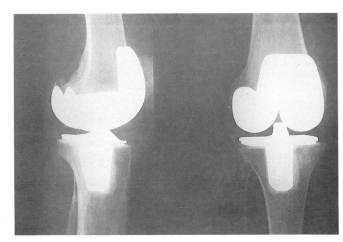

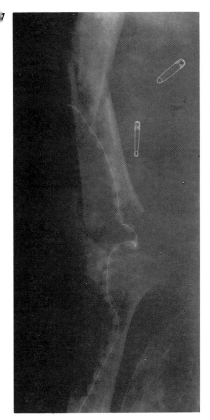

357 & 358 Complications of total knee arthroplasty in RA. Infection of an artificial joint remains one of the most serious complications of surgery. It may occasionally arise at the time of surgery, although this is much less common now that broad-spectrum prophylactic antibiotics are used peri-operatively. Delayed infection may occur, presumably from blood-borne organisms from an infected skin ulcer or possibly during dental work (*see* p.164). This patient with RA had an infected first prosthesis excised and replaced with a second fixed hinge, which again became infected. During the removal of this second hinge the femur was fractured. She spent 6 months in a splint with a flail knee, and antibiotic impregnated balls were inserted (**357**). At the third operation a specially made massive prosthesis was inserted (**358**). Six years later she developed a small discharging sinus at the lower pole of the incision and was prescribed regular antbiotics. She remained largely pain-free and was able to bear weight on this knee despite the chronic infection.

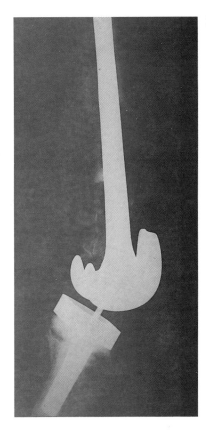

359

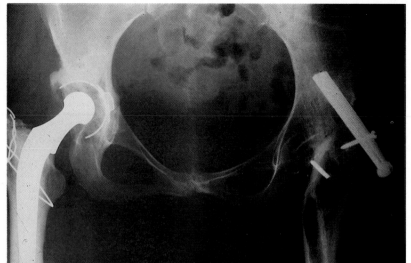

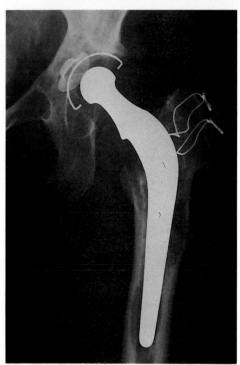

360

359 Arthroplasty of the hip. This patient, with OA of the hips due to undetected congenital dislocations, developed symptoms in her left hip in the early 1960s. With replacement arthroplasty still in its infancy at that time, she underwent the then standard procedure of hip fusion. This relieved the pain, but was very disabling, making sitting and standing up awkward. Ten years later, when the right hip became painful, she underwent a standard replacement arthroplasty, which remains satisfactory. She is now being considered for reconstruction and replacement of the fused hip in an attempt to relieve the strain on her lower lumbar spine.

360 Loosening of a total hip replacement. The weakest points of any weight-bearing prosthetic joint lie at the interfaces between bone and cement, and cement and prosthesis. Cement-free prostheses, coated with hydroxyapatite, are being used as a possible means of getting around this problem, but their long-term benefit has yet to be proven. This X-ray demonstrates radiolucent areas of bone resorption. The resorption is seen adjacent to the stem of the prosthesis and is thought to be induced by particulate matter derived from the prosthesis, which is forced (under the pressure of weight-bearing) down small fault channels which occur in the cement, especially at its interface with the prosthesis. The patient's hip was becoming increasingly painful and a second, cementless replacement was inserted successfully. No infection was found in this case.

Antibiotic prophylaxis in patients with indwelling artificial joints.

Wherever possible the risk of infection must be avoided in patients who have indwelling artificial joints; skin commensal organisms are the main cause of delayed infection. Ulceration of the skin, for whatever reason, and especially over prominent metatarsal heads in a forefoot affected by RA (*see* **35**), should be avoided by careful attention to pressure points. If ulceration occurs, it should be treated promptly and, if the ulcer becomes infected, antibiotic treatment should be given immediately. It is not clear whether patients with indwelling artificial joints are at risk of blood-borne infection during dental procedures, but prophylactic antibiotics are not generally advised for routine use, as the slight risk of serious side-effects from the antibiotics is probably higher than the risk of the replaced joint becoming infected.

12 Aids for the disabled

Arthritis and some of the other rheumatic disorders described in this book may lead to moderate or severe disability, which can be temporary or permanent. It is essential that the doctor and other health care professionals understand that the disabled person has rights that may require protection in a society which is, if not hostile, at least indifferent to the disabled.

Although drugs and surgery improve the individual's quality of life and may delay or reduce damage, many patients will greatly benefit from a variety of aids; some are cheap and simple but effective, whereas others are more costly and complex and need careful assessment. The best way to measure the individual's needs is by means of a formal functional assessment of mobility and of daily activities such as preparing and eating food, toileting and bathing, and dressing. A doctor or an occupational therapist will often need to visit the person in their home in order to assess them fully. It is also essential to consider the degree of social support that an individual enjoys from family, friends and social security agencies, all of whom may need to be involved in the discussion and decision making. The level of assistance needed will depend on the degree of disability, the amount of support available from others, and the type of accommodation in which the disabled person lives.

General mobility and access to transport is even more essential to the disabled person with arthritis than to the able bodied. Normal public transport remains woefully inadequate for the needs of the disabled in most countries. If finances are available, an automatic car with power steering can often be adapted to the needs of even the most severely disabled, and there are special driving and technical services available to assess the individual's needs. Any newly disabled person, or someone with progressive arthritis who cannot drive, should be encouraged to learn if at all possible. Alternatively, a wheelchair, hand propelled by the disabled person, or by a fit friend or relative or, in some circumstances, electrically driven, enables anyone with painful lower limb arthritis or other limitations to mobility to escape from an otherwise housebound existence and to achieve some degree of independence. Although there are signs of an increasing sensitivity to the needs of the disabled, access for wheelchair-bound people to public places remains inadequate.

Once disability has developed, it is the duty of the doctor and other members of the care team to assess the ways in which patients can be helped to cope better. Whether it is the provision of a walking stick of the correct length, or of simple aids to help in the performance of day-to-day activities (together with instruction on how to use them), the ordering of the most appropriate wheelchair for their needs, or the installation of a bath hoist or stair lift, the first step is to identify the need and then to meet it as well as the available resources permit.

Seating

361 Seating. Inappropriate seating is the bane of the day-to-day life of any person disabled by painful or weak hips. The correct height and depth of the seat are essential and must be appropriate to the individual: in general a higher than average seat is necessary. This correct height, together with firm arm rests, aids rising and sitting. For more severe cases, mechanical or electrically driven elevator chairs are available. Their action, which must be gentle, lifts the person to a standing position without toppling them over.

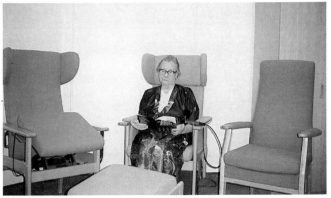

Mobility

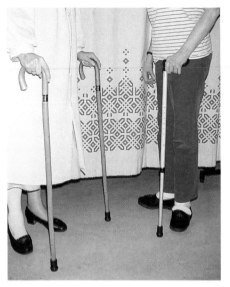

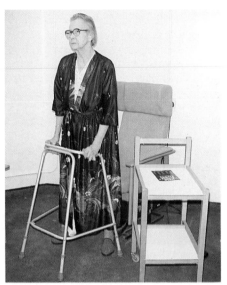

362 Walking sticks. Although many people feel there is a stigma attached to using a walking stick, once they can be persuaded to try one they often agree that it is helpful not only as a means of partial weight displacement to the upper limb (this is generally best achieved with the stick in the hand opposite to the more severely affected leg), but also as an aid to stability (a tripod stick may be more helpful) and, last but not least, as a warning to others to be thoughtful. The stick should be of the correct length and of a type suited to the patient's need and hand function. A folding stick is convenient and appropriate for some.

Any form of walking aid effectively transfers some weight-bearing function to the upper limb. This should be borne in mind when the upper limbs are also affected.

363 Walking frames. A variety of walking frames is available including folding models and those that are waist height or higher, with gutter attachments allowing weight-bearing through the forearms and sparing the hands. Some can be fitted with a carrying bag or tray, which goes some way towards compensating patients for the inevitable loss of freedom to use the hands.

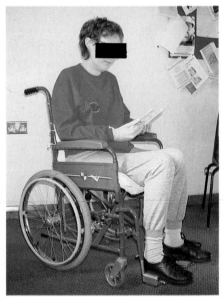

364 Wheelchairs. The choice of wheelchair is an expert function and any patient in need of one should seek advice from an appropriate therapist. Not only must the patient's size and weight be assessed, but also their more specific requirements of the chair. The home and working environment must also be inspected before a decision is made. Door widths, the height of beds and toilets (for transferring to and from the chair) and that of working surfaces, together with the provision of adequate knee space under them, all need to be considered. It may be necessary to convert steps to ramps, both indoors and out. Most disabled people prefer to remain in their familiar home surroundings, which can be adapted in a variety of different ways. However, it is sometimes advisable for them to move into accommodation that is specially adapted for wheelchair occupants.

Different types of wheelchair are available, answering different needs. A lightweight, folding chair will permit stowing in the boot of a car, but the car size must be adequate. Chairs can be self-propelled if upper limb function is satisfactory, pushed by an assistant (assuming that one is available) or electrically driven. A battery-driven chair is an expensive purchase, requiring careful choice of the most appropriate model. Patients and their relatives should be clear that the choice is appropriate and the expense justified. In some countries all such chairs are available and financed through special schemes for the disabled.

Driving for the disabled

As mobility and independence are of paramount importance to most people with disabling diseases, if it can be afforded, a car is seen as essential to many. The car can be adapted to suit the individual whether as a driver or as a passenger. A special driving centre for the disabled is the ideal place both to decide on the best make of car and the adaptations needed, and to teach the person to drive again. As the modifications can be expensive, all disabled drivers should be urged to seek expert advice before they purchase a car.

Food preparation and eating

365–367 A selection of kitchen aids. The range of aids for use in the home is enormous. Some are readily available and not made specifically for the disabled. An electric can-opener, a lightweight whisk, lightweight double-handed saucepans fitted with sieves into which food can be placed (thus avoiding the need to lift heavy pans of hot water) are a few examples. For those with poor hand function, large-handled lightweight knives, kettle tippers and devices to hold articles in place are available. Taps and electrical plugs can be adapted to make them easier to handle. Guidance should be sought through what can appear to be a maze of alternatives. As important as the devices themselves are the heights of surfaces and cupboards and the provision of a perching stool or other appropriate seat.

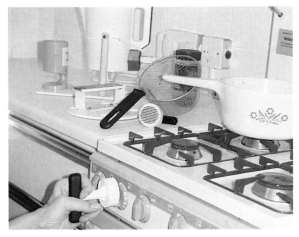

365

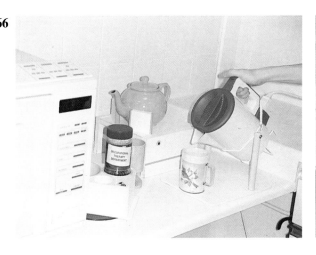

366

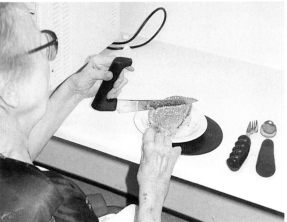

367

Personal hygiene and dressing

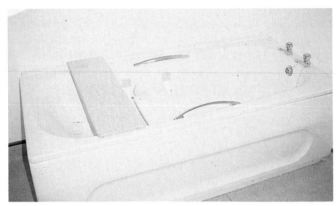

368–370 Bath aids. A variety of different aids is available to enable the disabled to enjoy a soak in the bath. These range from a simple bath board, through a variety of self-operated rise and fall seats, to floor- or ceiling-mounted hoists. Chosen with care they can increase independence and/or reduce the risks to both patient and carer. A walk-in shower, without a lip or step, and a plastic chair to sit in during showering may be more appropriate for some.

369

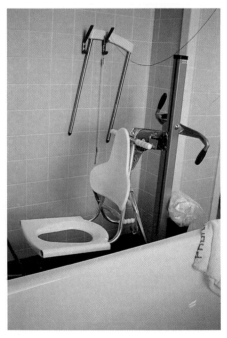

370

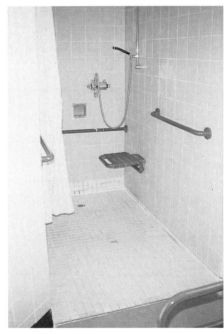

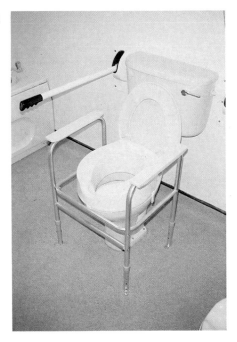

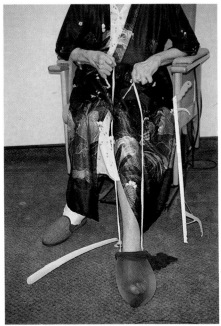

371 Use of the toilet. A raised toilet pedestal or a raised seat to place over the toilet make independent use of the toilet safer and preserve privacy, which most prefer. Fixed railings around the toilet are also helpful. For the severely disabled living alone, units are available which use warm water and air to wash and dry at the press of a button.

372 Dressing aids. It may be necessary to choose clothes that are loose fitting, with limited numbers of awkward fastenings. For day-to-day use, many disabled people find that track suits are ideal. Front-fastening clothing with zips or velcro rather than buttons is suitable and worth looking for. It need not be unfashionable! When unmodified clothes are desired, a variety of dressing aids may be of help, for example, button hooks, dressing sticks, and aids to put on stockings or socks.

Shoes for the disabled

Although it is not inevitable, most shoes that are made to fit deformed feet do not conform with modern fashions. Broad fittings with an adequate toe box are comfortable and protect pressure points. The soles should be lightweight but thick and shock-absorbent. For indoor use a pair of training shoes with a velcro fastening can be helpful. However, it is a pity that most manufacturers do not make such footwear in colours and styles more suitable for the older person. Off-the-peg shoes for difficult feet are available from some retail outlets. Shoes that are handmade from specially formed lasts are extremely expensive, requiring expert (and preferably independent) advice before being purchased.

Security

In these days of increasing crime it is important to remember that the disabled are extremely vulnerable to attacks upon their person and their property. If they are attacked or if they fall, they may need to be able to contact someone urgently. Personal security alarms in the form of a bracelet or pendant that connects to an ordinary or a voice-activated telephone can greatly reduce the risk. Access to the home must be secure, but there should be a reliable keyholder nearby in case of an accident. Remote-control door locks provide effective control over access, with a voice or televisual link to the street making it possible to check the identity of callers prior to their admission.

For the more severely disabled, it may be necessary to consider other options, for example, electrically or mechanically elevating chairs, and electrically operated beds, stair lifts or hoists. The wide selection of aids available for the disabled is beyond the scope of this book.

The inevitable limitation for many patients is the availability of funds to pay for equipment. Social services or charities may help. The battle for the proper provision of such aids to independent living is well worth fighting. In many countries, there are now patient self-help groups and voluntary advisory bodies, as well as resources available through social security and health care services. The doctor's surgery is an ideal place for information leaflets and contact addresses to be made available, and the health care professions have a duty provide this service.

INDEX

Figures in **bold** refer to illustrations.

hormone replacement therapy 131
humeral head, aseptic necrosis 41, **313**
hydralazine 10, 92
hydrocortisone hemisuccinate 20, **15**
hydroxychloroquine 48 (table), 97
hypercholesterolaemia, familial 143,
    317–318
hypermobility syndrome 10, 135,
    300–301
hyperparathyroidism 130
hypertrophic (pulmonary)
    osteoarthropathy (HPOA) 140
hyperuricaemia 59, 60 (table), 63
hypopyon 82, **192**
hypothyroidism 130, **288**

IgG rheumatoid factors 16, **3**
immune complex deposition 39, **86, 89**
indomethacin 62, 63 (table)
industrial injury 10
infection risk with indwelling artificial
    joints 164
infective arthritis 9, 33, **64–65,** 126
infective endocarditis 9
inflammatory arthritis 49
    feet 24, **31–32**
    management 157
interstitial fibrosing alveolitis 41, **95**
iridocyclitis 118, 119, **267**
irritable bowel syndrome 155
isoniazid 92

jaw in polyarticular-onset juvenile
    chronic arthritis 117, **261**
joint
    arthroplasty 57
    artificial indwelling 164
    aspiration equipment 146, **323**
    destruction 139
    effusion in reactive arthritis 88, **209**
    movement 11
juvenile chronic arthritis 113
    generalised growth retardation 116,
    260
    management 119
    pauciarticular-onset 118–19
    polyarticular-onset 115–17
    systemic-onset 113 (table), 114,
    252–255

keratoconjunctivitis sicca 42, **97**
keratoderma blenorrhagica 87, **205**
kidney
    amyloid deposits in rheumatoid
    arthritis 46, **112–113**
    involvement in systemic sclerosis
    102, **237,** 103
kitchen aids 167, **365–367**

Klebsiella spp. 77, 83
knee
    acromegalic 129, **286**
    arthroplasty 162, **354–358**
    aspiration 27, **44,** 153, **341**
    chondrocalcinosis 64, **152–3**
    in FMF 143
    gonococcal arthritis 126, **277**
    local injection techniques 153,
    341–342
    medial ligament pain 153, **342**
    metaphyseal overgrowth in juvenile
    polyarthritis 117, **262**
    monarthritis in Crohn's disease 90,
    212
    osteoarthritis 49, **115,** 53, **128–131**
    osteotomy 159, **346–347**
    rheumatoid arthritis in 26, **38–52**
    synovectomy 158
    synovitis 26, **38**
    tabes dorsalis 139
    total replacement 29, **50–52,** 159
    traumatic lesions 123, **270–273**
    valgus 28, **47,** 28, **49,** 29, **50–52**
    varus 29, **50–52**

latex agglutination test 15, **2**
lead poisoning 59
leg ulceration 38, **83**
limbs, examination 11
lipid
    metabolism disorders 143
    storage disease 143
livedo reticularis 109, **247**
local injection techniques 145–154
    complications 145
    elbow 147, **324–325,** 148, **326–327**
    equipment 146, **323**
    heel 154, **344**
    hip 154, **343**
    postinjection flare 145
    shoulder 148, **328–336**
    wrist 151, **337–340**
locomotor system examination 6, 9,
    10–12
loop diuretics 59
Looser's zones 132, **292**
low back pain management 76
lungs, interstitial disease 41, **95**
lupus band test 96, **224**
Lyme disease 128, **283**
lymphadenopathy 46, **114,** 137
lymphoedema 46, **114**
lymphoma 126, 127, **280–282**

malignancy, myositic presentation 9
Marfan's disease 135
medial meniscus tear 123, **270–272**
metacarpophalangeal (MCP) joint 19,
    13, 22, **25–27,** 32, **62**

metatarsophalangeal (MTP) joint 23,
    30–35
    acute gout 60, **141**
    hallux rigidus 53, **126–127**
methotrexate 39, **86,** 47, 48 (table), 86
methyldopa 92
micrognathia 117, **261**
mixed connective tissue disease
    (MCTD) 108
mobility 165
monarthritis 9
mononeuritis multiplex 45, **109**
monosodium urate 59, 60, **140**
muscle
    fibrosis 104
    paraspinal wasting in AS 79,
    182–184
    spasm 67, 68, **159**
myelomatosis 142
myopathy, corticosteroid-induced 107
myxoedema 130, **288**

nail
    dystrophy 84, **196–197,** 87, **205**
    pitting 84, **195**
nail fold
    capillary abnormalities in
    dermatomyositis 106, **243**
    capillary changes in scleroderma
    98, **226**
    vasculitis 39, **86**
naproxen 62, 63 (table)
neck pain 68, **159**
nephrotic syndrome 46, **110–111**
nerve
    entrapment 44
    root compression 69 (table),
    161–162, 75 (table)
neuropathic arthritis 138–9
neuropathy, bilateral peripheral sensory
    45, **108**
nifedipine 94, **218,** 103
non-steroidal anti-inflammatory drugs
    (NSAIDs)
    in acute pseudogout 66
    in AS 83
    in gout 62, 63 (table)
    in osteoarthritis 54, **130,** 54, **132,** 57
    in reactive arthritis 89
    renal side-effects 45
    in rheumatoid arthritis 47
    in SLE 97

occupational therapy 47, 57
ocular manifestations of rheumatoid
    arthritis 42, **97–105**
oesophagus in CREST syndrome 102,
    235
olecranon bursitis 31, **59,** 60, **142,** 61,
    143